W9-BSW-433

Getting a Jump on Fitness

Getting a Jump on Fitness

BARBARA MARROTT

BARRICADE BOOKS, INC. / New York

Published by Barricade Books Inc.
150 Fifth Avenue
Suite 700
New York, NY 10011

Copyright © 1997 by Barbara Marrott

All rights reserved.

No part of this book may be reproduced, stored in a retrieval system, or transmitted in any form, by any means, including mechanical, electronic, photocopying, recording, or otherwise, without the prior written permission of the publisher, except by a reviewer who wishes to quote brief passages in connection with a review written for inclusion in a magazine, newspaper, or broadcast.

Printed in the United States of America.
Book design by Cindy LaBreacht.
Cover and all interior photographs by Robert Milazzo.
Hair and makeup by Christina Liberatore.

Library of Congress Cataloging-in-Publication Data

Marrott, Barbara.
    Getting a jump on fitness / Barbara Marrott.
        p.   cm.
    ISBN 1-56980-102-9
    1. Rope skipping. 2. Physical fitness. I. Title.
GV498.M36   1997
796.2—dc21   96-49159
                                              CIP

10 9 8 7 6 5 4 3 2 1

ACKNOWLEDGMENTS

I would like to thank my 6:30 A.M., dedicated, and loyal students, not only for their commitment to fitness, but also for their commitment to me. The group has grown rapidly, and many of them have been with me for nearly ten years, following me to take classes wherever I teach. Because of their open-mindedness and their enthusiasm in embracing anything I throw their way, they allow me to reach new heights in my creativity. These people are not professional athletes, but rather regular working people and housewives, who are truly devoted to good health and fitness.

I want to thank photographer extraordinaire, Robert Milazzo, who not only is an exceptionally talented and creative photographer, but is also a true pleasure with whom to be affiliated. Another phenomenal artist is Christina Liberatore, whose skilled hands and talented vision make her a supreme hair and makeup artist, with effervescence and class. To both Robert and Christina, I give my deepest gratitude (especially for balancing that fine line between glamorous photos and grassroots fitness, so much so, that my students and clients may roll their eyes and say, "She NEVER looks like that when she teaches!").

Thanks to Lorraine and Chloe, my generous, faithful, and talented jumpers!

Thank you to Carole Stuart and Lisa Beck at Barricade Books for believing in this project, and to Sandy Stuart for her skilled comments and careful eye.

Of course, none of this would be possible without the love and support of my husband, Bruce, and my daughter, Lauren. Bruce made it possible for me to make a career change and do what I really love, in addition to having the patience while I jumped, stretched, and faxed my way through this book. It isn't just fitness that adds years to my life, but my daughter, Lauren, who gives me a million reasons to want to stay healthy.

And the most special thanks to my publicist and good friend, Rodi Rosensweig, whose support and guidance made this book possible. Her intelligence, logic, organization, creativity, humor, and ability to always turn something negative into positive is appreciated more than she'll ever know. She is a grounding force in my life.

Barbara Marrott
June 1997

TABLE OF CONTENTS

MY OUTLOOK ON FITNESS

Three years ago, I went to a seminar on youth fitness. The seminar focused on an array of fitness-related activities for children. We played games like duck-duck goose, dodge ball, and other gym-class staples. My memories of elementary school came rushing back. I remembered that being a naturally athletic person, I got picked first for teams, and, in many cases, I was chosen captain. My best friend, however, was considered "chubby," and she was chosen last on a team just to "even it up."

Unfortunately, we are stamped with negative feelings toward fitness abilities at a very young age. Those feelings stay with us throughout adulthood. With a little luck, someone or something helps us to realize how wrong we were.

Let's take the game duck-duck goose. Everyone sits in a circle, and one individual is chosen to walk around that circle tapping each person while saying "duck, duck" and so on until he or she chooses a "goose." The goose has to get up as quickly as possible and run after the person who tapped him. Think about it. Are most children likely to choose the fastest person in the class? How about the second fastest? In most cases, the answer is "no." In my opinion, this game encourages people to pick on the slower runner or the less-athletic individual.

Dodge ball is another one of those games. The class gets divided into two teams. A line of rubber balls divides the two sides down the middle. When the whistle blows, each side runs to pick up one of the balls to throw at someone on the opposing team. Sound like fun? I hated this class. My stomach got in a big knot, and my heart pounded. (Pretty serious comment for someone who was voted the most athletic girl in school.) It finally dawned on me why the first thing so many of my clients say to me is "I haven't exercised since I was a kid. I am not coordinated. I was never good in gym class. I am not the athletic type. I always hated gym class . . . " No matter what age (my clients range from nine to seventy), they make a direct correlation between their gym-class memory and their physical abilities. Frankly, I don't understand what being hit by a dodge ball has to do with someone's physical fitness level, ability, and coordination.

As a certified fitness practitioner, personal trainer, and aerobics instructor, I have come across all body types, ages, athletic abilities, and levels of coordination. With the exception of only two physically challenged people, every one of my clients have one thing in common: they all can jump rope. As a matter of fact, after a little practice, they all can jump rope VERY well. No matter how busy their lives are (some are high-powered executives, some full-time moms, some doctors and lawyers, some own small businesses), they have each found the answer to a quick, fun shot of true fitness—jumping rope. (It is important to note that their jump rope ability is not nearly as varied as their lives!)

I am completely convinced that, with the exception of certain medical conditions, everyone can jump rope and actually enjoy it. I made jumping rope part of my fitness program when I was thirty-one and became better at it as an adult than when I was a little girl at age ten, jumping outside with my friends in the schoolyard.

My Journey to This Book

Before I decided to write this book, I did a lot of research. First, I went to several prominent gyms in Manhattan with the idea of offering jump-rope classes. I was disappointed at the reactions that I received. The responses were completely unfounded. They ranged from "jump rope is bad for you" (see chapter 2 for my opinion and the medical fact on this one); "jump rope is not 'cutting edge' enough"; "the ceiling in the gym is too low"; "we have somebody who teaches boxing—which includes jumping"; "there isn't enough room for jumping. Since the jump rope takes up more space, we cannot pack as many people into the classes as we can in other classes . . . "

I interpreted their reactions as "this is new, and we don't know how to make it happen!" and "this might not generate as much income for the gym."

But, I held on to my proven research and professional fitness experience, the positive reaction I had received from my clients and classes, as well as the incredible results that I have seen from those who jump rope. I persevered in my research, and, it is my hope that this book will enable everyone to enjoy the benefits of jumping rope.

Since my meetings, several gyms have added jump-rope classes. This happened for two reasons: 1) boxing classes grew in popularity over the past two years, introducing people to the jump rope again. These people became aware of the cardiovascular demands from the jump-rope portion of those classes. And 2) the fitness industry was in dire need of something new. The industry evolves quickly, and the demand for new fitness trends and ideas is constant—first high-impact aerobics, then low-impact aerobics, then the step workouts, then the slide. You get the picture.

My research continued. I took a field trip to several bookstores to scan the shelves and see what kind of exercise books existed on the market. I asked one saleswoman which books sold the most and what it was that interested people in the fitness and health areas. Aside from the occasional celebrity fad book or success story, she said that there really was not very much out there that piqued and kept people's interest.

Our conversation continued with my asking her if she exercised. Her response was truly an eyeopener. She explained that she has three children and fell into the middle-income bracket. Her days are spent running her children to school and then to their other activities. When the kids are in school, that is her time to do housework, grocery shopping, and other errands. "I need a fitness plan that does not take a lot of time out of my life and that maybe I can do while my kids are in the park. I know many of the other mothers feel the same way. None of us can even take the time to get to a gym."

I started thinking more and more about how many people are stuck in this or similar situations, where fitness and exercise seem completely impossible to fit into their already stressful routines. Life gets in the way of health. I feel passionate about changing people's perception of the importance of fitness. Life IS health, but unfortunately, if we are pressured for time, the first thing we give up is exercise, mainly because we don't love it and it is a great way to rationalize getting out of it.

Stop for a moment and think about your routine. Would it be so horrible if the living room didn't get dusted until tomorrow because you took fifteen minutes to exercise today? How about not mopping the kitchen floor? Would anyone notice? How about getting up twenty minutes earlier? Would that twenty minutes truly exhaust you for the day? What about eating dinner twenty minutes later? Would your body adjust?

And, how about you—you, personally? Do you think that you would feel different about yourself if you took fifteen to twenty minutes, three or four times a week to exercise a little? YES, YOU WOULD! I promise you. I also guarantee you that your loved ones would be so busy noticing how happy and healthy you are that they would not have the time to notice what didn't get done in those few minutes each day.

I can promise that if you just exercise for fifteen minutes, it will give you a certain self-confidence that you have never had before. It will relieve stress better than any medication, and you will really be better at everything you do, simply because you will be a happier, more confident person.

This goes for both women and men. Exercise is not a luxury. It is a *necessity*. It is a vital part of personal hygiene, and it should be taught that way. Could you imagine not brushing your teeth? Your teeth would turn slimy green, be filled with cavities, and eventually fall out. Sound appealing? Well, what if your bones got holes in them and broke because they were so brittle? What if you became so overweight and unhealthy that you could not stand to look at yourself in the mirror? What about the increased risk of heart attack and stroke? Is it worth omitting exercise from your life?

Granted, brushing your teeth is a lot quicker, but it is certainly not any more of a necessity.

Look at exercise as an investment in your future. You want to continue to be able to do things for your partner, your children, and your children's children.

Ready?

Now that I have told you my philosophy of exercise and health, I will show you how to incorporate exercise into your life. It is possible. And, believe it or not, this is a fun, easy, exciting, unique, and effective way to get healthy.

CHAPTER 1

INTRODUCTION

How I Started

Every morning I teach a regular neighborhood class at 6:30 to a group of dedicated people who need a dose of exercise before facing the day. Their ages range from thirty to sixty years old.

After countless step routines and many body-sculpting classes, I was seeking variety in order to continually challenge my students and to keep them from getting bored. One day I got into my car and headed to an exercise equipment supply store looking for something—anything—that would give me creative inspiration. As I scrutinized the shelves, there it was, staring at me, saying "pick me!"—a perfect plastic jump rope.

The next morning, I passed around my new toys to the class. Everyone was buzzing. "Oh, I loved jumping rope when I was younger." "I haven't done this in so long." "I used to be great at this." Just taking the jump ropes in their hands brought big smiles to all of their faces. This added an entirely new dimension to my class.

I began by interspersing forty-five seconds of jumping rope in between a few minutes of stepping. After forty-five minutes of these "intervals" with the jumping and other exercises that they were already familiar with, my students were thrilled with their new workout. And, when my students are happy, I am very happy!

After six weeks, each student was given a new rope—one that was "weighted." The weighted plastic rope provides not only an aerobic workout, but also a full upper-body workout. This is due to the light, additional weight balanced in the rope. We began to gradually increase our jump rope intervals from forty-five seconds to ninety seconds in between our other exercises. Then we advanced to three minutes of jumping, and as time passed, our class was able to jump for five minutes. Soon, the class was jumping for even longer and began to experiment with various jumping patterns.

Finally, the day came when I said, "Don't set up your steps or other equipment. Everyone, just take out your ropes." My students expect the unexpected from me, yet it was with great skepticism that they took out their ropes. After our warmup, I told them we were jumping for seven minutes. To their surprise, that was not so bad. Then I said, "Let's try another seven minutes." As we worked toward a goal of increased endurance, within six months my class was jumping rope twice a week for thirty minutes straight and performing various tricks while jumping.

The jump rope gave birth to many other types of classes. One of my favorites (and theirs, too) is taking the class and their ropes outside for workouts. You can't beat that! It is definitely an eyeopener at 6:30 in the morning.

The point of my sharing this story with you is that these are regular people who learned how to jump rope well, while enjoying the rope for its versatility. It is important to note that I do not claim to be the world's greatest jump roper. I have not won any competitions, broken any records, or by any stretch of the imagination, mastered all of the tricks. This book is not about fancy footwork or tricks. It is about a basic, fun, creative, and successful approach to exercise.

By using the methods described here, I have added variety to my clients' and students' workouts and exercise programs. I have also taught them something quite enlightening: they are probably better at jump rope as an adult than they ever were as children (which, incidentally, is an incredible confidence booster). More importantly, this has opened people's eyes. There is an alternative for those who are pressed for time or hate going to the gym or come up with a number of reasons for giving up exercise. Every one of the workouts that I will share with you can be done indoors or out, in a big house or small apartment, with little or no equipment except for a jump rope.

If this book, and jumping rope, inspires an individual who is not currently exercising to actually get up off of the couch and say, "You know what? This sounds pretty good. I think I'll give it a try," then I will feel successful.

What Is Physical Fitness?

Physical fitness has different meanings for different people. It is not limited to Olympic medalists, marathon runners, or triathletes. I refer to the term physical fitness as the capacity of the heart, blood vessels, lungs, and muscles to function at a high level of efficiency. A person who is physically fit has an enhanced functional capacity that allows for a higher quality of life—that is, an overall positive feeling and enthusiasm for life. It is the ability to perform routine and required activities without fatigue and exhaustion. By doing so, the individual is then able to participate in additional pleasurable activities.

There are five major components of physical fitness:

1) MUSCULAR STRENGTH—the maximal force a muscle or muscle group can exert during contraction.

2) MUSCULAR ENDURANCE—the ability of a muscle or muscle group to exert a force against a resistance over a sustained period of time. An example of this would be the number of times you can lift a specified weight before experiencing fatigue.

3) CARDIOVASCULAR (CARDIORESPIRATORY) ENDURANCE—many people refer to this as aerobic fitness. This is the capacity of the heart, lungs, and blood vessels to deliver nutrients and oxygen to the working muscles and tissues during sustained exercise. Metabolic waste and other products that would result in fatigue are also removed. By performing a regular, moderately intense program of aerobic exercise, one may maintain an efficient cardiorespiratory system.

4) FLEXIBILITY—an adequate degree of flexibility is achieved when you are able to move your joints through a normal full-range of motion. Flexibility prevents injury and allows us to stay mobile.

5) BODY COMPOSITION—body composition is broken down into two parts: lean body mass and body fat. Lean body mass consists of muscles, bones, nervous tissue, skin, blood, and organs. Because these tissues are metabolically very active, they contribute to energy production during exercise. Body fat, otherwise known as adipose tissue, is that component of the body responsible for storing energy for later use. Some body fat is essential in order to maintain normal bodily functions. This body fat is called essential body fat. Women must maintain between 8 and 12 percent body fat of their total body weight. Falling below this percentage can affect one's reproductive system. In many cases, a women will cease to have her menstrual cycle. This is known as amenorrhea. Subcutaneous fat is the fat most of us want to rid ourselves of. This type of fat is found stored under the skin and found deep inside the body. A large amount of this type of fat is known as obesity.

Muscular strength and muscular endurance are achieved through resistive training (weightlifting and calisthenic exercises). Many people ignore this aspect in fitness. Women in particular think that they will "bulk up" when they lift weights. However, if done correctly, this cannot happen. Instead, when done properly, and you are not fanatical about lifting, healthy muscular definition occurs. Lifting weights two or three times a week is simply restoring muscle that has been lost. Resistance training is a great antiaging exercise. In addition, it maintains muscle tone, prevents osteoporosis, builds strength, and, yes, it burns calories! As a matter of fact, it has a longer lasting effect on calorie burning than riding the exercise bike, jogging on the treadmill, or doing the StairMaster for the same amount of time.

Weight training accomplishes this by building muscle mass. I hope you are not thinking of the "Gladiators" because that is not the type of muscle building I am talking about. I am talking about Elle MacPhersonish muscle tone. (That conjures up a better picture for you, doesn't it?)

Between our twenties and thirties, we lose muscle mass. In this age range, this loss is preventable through weightlifting. Not fifteen-, twenty-, or thirty-five-pound weights. I am talking about three-, five-, and eight-pound weights. Part of the aging process involves a decrease in the number of muscle cells. However, through weight training, one can increase the size and strength of the cells. The loss of muscle results in other changes, as well. You may weigh the same, but your body shape can change and your metabolism might slow down because the less muscle you have, the less energy you burn at rest. I gained six pounds this year because I placed a greater emphasis on resistance training—but, I have never looked slimmer.

One of the great things about the workouts in this book is that they will provide you with workouts that include resistive training either through exercises like lunges and squats; household items as substitutes for exercise equipment; and, of course, my favorite tool in the world, the beloved jump rope.

What Is My Heart Rate?

I will often refer to your heart rate when doing cardiovascular exercise. You may wonder, "what is it and what does it really mean?"

Your heart rate is simply the number of times that your heart beats per minute. For example, let's say you take your heart rate, and you learn that it beats seventy-two times in one minute. Now what? What does that mean?

To give you a benchmark, a marathon runner or athlete's heart rate may be as low as fifty beats per minute. Your heart is a muscle, and its function is to pump blood throughout your body. It becomes stronger through exercise. As it gains in strength, it is capable of pumping more blood in a single beat than it was before. Therefore, if it had to pump seventy-two times in one minute to send out a given amount of blood before embarking on an exercise program, it may only have to pump or beat sixty-four times to send out the same amount of blood after following an exercise program because you strengthened the heart muscle. In simple terms, your heart does not have to work as hard to pump out the same amount of blood in a given time.

Factors that affect your heart rate are:

1) HIGH CHOLESTEROL OR CLOGGED ARTERIES. With this condition, your heart has to work extra hard to pump blood past fat globules to get where it has to go.

2) SMOKING. If you smoke, then your heart rate will be increased, and your lungs will get clogged from the nicotine.

3) HIGH BLOOD PRESSURE (HYPERTENSION). This increases your heart rate. If you suffer from this, the blood that is pumped out by your heart exerts greater pressure on the walls of your arteries.

The list goes on and on!

Remember when we talked about personal hygiene, and I said that exercise was not a luxury? Exercise falls into the category of self-preservation. It takes about fifteen minutes longer than it takes to brush your teeth, but you don't have to do it twice a day. The American College of Sports Medicine recommends exercising three times a week for about twenty minutes. That works out to about nine minutes a day! Most of us spend more time than that blow-drying our hair!

How Do I Find Out What My Heart Rate Is?

Let me make it clear that before embarking on any exercise program, I strongly advise that you get your physician's approval. This is especially true if you are taking any medications or if you have not had a physical in the past year.

Here is how you figure out what your heart rate should be while exercising.

AGE-PREDICTED MAXIMAL HEART RATE
1) Start with the number 220.
2) Subtract your age.

Keep in mind that this number is only an estimate and can vary by as much as twenty-four beats per minute. A thirty-five-year-old woman can vary from 161 to 185 beats per minute while she's exercising.

TALK TEST FOR HEART RATE This is exactly what it says. You should be able to talk during exercise. You should not be gasping for air. You should not be feeling dizzy, light headed, or nauseous. If you feel your heart pounding, walk until it slows down. Do not sit down! Listen to your body. It can tell you so much.

Interval Circuit Training

Because the jump rope is so cardiovascularly demanding, I have found that the best way to build stamina is to use intervals and circuits or "interval circuit training," a term I will use many times throughout this book. Interval and circuit training have been around for many years, and they are workout styles that improve aerobic and anaerobic conditioning. I combine the two for my clients and students and for the workouts in this book.

Interval training alternates periods of work and rest. A lower-intensity rest period follows a high-intensity work period. By using the interval training method, an individual can produce more work in a given time if the work is spaced between periods of rest.

For example, a professional athlete may be able to exercise at his or her peak intensity for twelve minutes before becoming too exhausted to continue. However, if the athlete were to break up the twelve minutes into intervals, it would look something like this:

- 3 minutes of jumping rope
- 3 minutes of walking
- 3 minutes of jumping rope
- 3 minutes of walking
- 3 minutes of jumping rope
- 3 minutes of walking
- 3 minutes of jumping rope
- 3 minutes of walking.

With this workout, the athlete would be able to work for twenty-four minutes before experiencing the same degree of fatigue that would occur in twelve minutes.

There are many advantages to interval training, some of which are not relative to this book. But, here are some that you should keep in mind when going through the workouts in the following chapters.

1) Interval training provides variety and therefore prevents boredom.

2) It generally causes fewer injuries due to the varied intensity.

3) It provides greater potential for a greater total workout.

4) It improves aerobic and anaerobic power and capacity.

5) It increases exercise adherence.

What if you can only jump rope for thirty seconds? Here is what you could do.

- Jump for 15 seconds.
- Walk for 15 seconds.

- Jump for 15 seconds.
- Walk for 15 seconds.

You just doubled your workout time. Eventually you will be able to jump for one minute before fatigue sets in and so on. This is a GREAT way to start!

On the other hand, circuit training means that a person moves from one "station" to the next with little (fifteen to thirty seconds) or no rest, performing a fifteen- to forty-five-second workout of eight to twenty repetitions before experiencing fatigue.

For the purpose of this book, no machines will be used, and the focus is on interval circuit training (the combination of both styles). You do not need machines to get in shape. Instead, I will teach you how to use a combination of the jump rope (for jumping, stretching, and resistance) as well as bands, lunges, squats, and the option of free weights. (You may fill bottles with water or sand to reach a desired weight. Throughout this book, I interchange bottles and weights.) By adding these other exercises between each jumping rope segment, this type of training can improve cardiorespiratory and muscular endurance.

The concept of interval circuit training is used by both professionals and beginners. It has gotten a very positive response from the professional health and fitness community since it takes the focus off the actual exercises and, instead, makes the process and variations the point of the workout. By focusing on changing what you are doing every couple of minutes, you won't get bored and won't think about what fatigues you, because in minutes, you will be doing a different exercise.

With an interval circuit program using the jump rope and the workouts in this book, YOU WILL NOT be bored, exhausted, or get frustrated. YOU CAN DO IT!

Why Should You Exercise?

Okay, you know that I believe in the mental and physical benefits of interval circuit training, and I strongly advise you to give it a try.

There is something very important I want you to know.

It is much better to prevent a problem than to treat one. When it comes to your health and your body, there are three steps that you can take to prevent health problems. 1) Avoid undue risk factors (i.e. smoking, excessive alcohol, unsafe sex, recreational drugs, etc.). 2) Eat sensibly (consume a nutritionally sound diet). 3) Exercise regularly.

I want you to live a long, healthy life, and if exercise can make that happen . . . well, you decide.

Undoubtedly, you have heard over and over again many good reasons for exercising. But just in case you missed some, here are some other reasons regular exercise should be a part of your life.

EXERCISING:

1) Helps the body resist upper respiratory tract infections;

2) Reduces risk of developing high blood pressure;

3) Increases circulating levels of HDL cholesterol (the good kind);

4) Helps improve short-term memory (especially in older people);

5) Assists in efforts to stop smoking;

6) Enhances sexual desire, performance, and satisfaction;

7) Improves posture;

8) Helps relieve headaches;

9) Helps relieve many of the common discomforts of pregnancy;

10) Helps reduce anxiety and depression.

Pretty good stuff, huh? Don't take my word for it. Give it a try.

CHAPTER 2

MY FAVORITE TOOL AND EVERYTHING YOU EVER WANTED TO KNOW ABOUT THE JUMP ROPE

The History of Jump Rope

Like so many ancient games, sports, and rituals, the origin of the jump rope is unclear. What is known is that thousands of years ago, our ancestors began to make games out of the skills that were essential to their survival. Running, leaping, and throwing were of vital importance to primitive hunters, and, therefore, it can be concluded that children watched and imitated their elders (as they always do). As the children mimicked the adults, survival techniques evolved into games. Such skills slowly became formalized and, by the time of the ancient Greeks, athletic sports had become an important part of life—for both children and adults.

The first jumping games seemed to have involved contests where children competed in jumping and leaping across a stream or over a rock. Thousands of years later, vines or some other fibrous material (Spaniards used leather thongs, Hungarians used straw) were used as a "bar" to leap over. While this is conjecture, it is certain that rope-jumping games were played in most every country of the world with similar evolution.

Jumping over the "bar," or rope, eventually found its way to the actual activity of jumping or skipping rope (quite similar to the way we know it today). This seems likely to have had its origins in ancient Egypt and China when ropemakers actually jumped over their ropes by turning them upwards, over their heads, to pick up loose hemp strands. As children watched, they began to imitate the jumping and, just like jumping over rocks and skipping around trees, jumping over the rope in this fashion (overhead) became another jumping game. By this point, some were using ropes, "sash" cords from window pulls and other various cords, or anything else that would serve the same purpose. In Sweden, they used stiff wicker. French children played with string ropes woven on spool looms. Cherokee Indians used wild grapevines. Kids in New Zealand used cow ropes. And in England, the bobbin spindles of mill-weaving machine were converted into handles at the ends of the ropes.

Sailors exported these ideas through their travels around the world. From simple singular jumping with the rope came some of the jump rope games we know today. These games were probably introduced to this country in the mid-1600s by Dutch settlers of New Amsterdam. However, for some reason, it was considered a boy's activity (probably with its origins and connections to male hunters using rope), especially in Western cultures. It's also interesting that as this boy's game became popular and girls wanted to participate, young girls were warned not to take part in such strenuous activities because their blood vessels would burst. (Hasn't exercise and games come a long way since then?) Of course, it was not long before women realized that this was an old wives' tale, and they began to jump, too. As the games involving jump rope multiplied and became increasingly popular, so did various chants and rhymes that went along with the games. Since the beat of the rope to the ground was rhythmic, it became a tradition to sing songs to the beat.

Jump rope (with boys and girls) became one of the most popular children's games in history. It was flexible, fun, and universal. You could have one, two, or several players. The rope was inexpensive. And it could be done virtually any place, any time. But the image somehow changed and, ironically, in the United States by the 1960s, rope jumping became a favorite activity for girls, and the boys who participated were called "sissies." Little girls singing and jumping alone or in groups could be seen in almost every schoolyard and playground.

Meanwhile, professional boxers (call them sissies!) have long recognized the incredible training properties of the jump rope, and was a crucial part of their exercise program. Prizefighters used the technique of single-rope skipping to help develop their lungs, legs, and coordination. It was apparent that basic jumping with a rope built coordination and skill, as well as balance and endurance, while also conditioning the heart and lungs and toning muscles in the upper and lower body.

Why should prizefighters and children get all of the benefits? Imagine, building coordination, balance, and endurance while toning muscles and actually HAVING FUN! Well, read on, and you will see how jumping rope can change your life.

Common Myths—Physical and Emotional— About Jumping Rope

Before I became a trained and certified fitness trainer and instructor, I believed people with bad backs and other medical conditions were unable to exercise aerobically. As I entered the fitness world on a professional level, I realized that certain exercise activities carry a negative image, especially jumping rope. People think that it is "not good for you." There are four popular—but inaccurate—perceptions about jumping rope (and many other aerobic activities). They are: people cannot jump if they have a bad back; jumping will destroy your knees; if you are not coordinated, you cannot jump rope; if you jump rope, you will get too winded.

Of the four, the first two may very well be legitimate for some people. But the other two are not. Jumping rope is a learned activity, and endurance is something that you build over time.

First, let's talk about a "bad back." If you are afraid to jump rope because you have a bad back, consider why you have a bad back. If you have never had an actual injury to your back or have never been diagnosed with a problem in your spine, take a look down your body, and focus on your abdomen. Most people refer to it as their stomach.

Your stomach is an organ, and it is responsible for storing, diluting, and digesting food. So, if you are one of those people who pat your hand on your abdomen and say, "I need to work on my stomach," go eat a sandwich. On the other hand, if you want to "tighten" your abdominal area, then you need to work on your abdominals. Your abdominals are muscles (stomach=organ; abs=muscle) and CAN BE tightened through exercise.

Now you may ask what does this has to do with a "bad back"? Well, when an individual gains weight, his or her spine is greatly affected because the spine holds up the body. As the abdominal area gets bigger, there is an exaggerated curve on the lower back. In addition, if you do not stay flexible and don't take the time to stretch daily, then the back of your legs (the hamstrings) tighten up. Since the hamstrings insert at the buttocks and at the lower back areas, when the legs are tight, this may cause back pain. The good news is that this problem can be corrected (and avoided) by strengthening your abdominals, as well as stretching not only the back, but also the legs, specifically the hamstrings.

Your first course of action in strengthening your back is to start watching your caloric intake so you lose weight. Next add light exercise like walking and gentle stretching. Very soon you will begin to relieve your back from the pressure by losing weight and stretching in the process. Your body will tell you when you are ready for the next step, which is to begin a workout program using the jump rope.

Remember: the jump rope will not CAUSE back injury. If you have a healthy, strong back (or want to have one by taking my above advice), then jumping rope will not hurt you.

Now, let's talk about bad knees. This is very similar to what I just explained about your back. The knees are bones. They are basically held in place by the muscles in the legs. Weak leg muscles place a great deal of stress on the knees. This is especially true for women with wide hips. Their knees may bother them because they feel the pressure of the wide hips, and when the leg muscles are not strong, the problem is worsened. The condition may be alleviated by strengthening the fronts of the upper legs known as the quadriceps, in addition to strengthening the outer thighs. On the other hand, if you had a recent knee-replacement procedure, I would not recommend a jump rope program.

Dr. Richard T. Braver is a sports podiatrist and team physician for Fairleigh Dickinson, Seton Hall, and Montclair State universities, as well as several professional teams. He points out that sports such as running do not involve full leg extension, which can cause an imbalance in the quadricep muscles surrounding the knee, leading to improper tracking of the kneecap. Jumping rope would complement running because of the full leg extension during push-offs. Dr. Braver is of the opinion that jumping rope can be an exhilarating and refreshing way to condition your body when done properly. So much for the belief that "jump rope is bad for you."

As for those who contend "I am not coordinated! I cannot jump rope!"—nonsense! Coordination is something that people can develop. With proper instruction, support, and confidence, which you can gain from this book, you will see that with a little patience and perseverance, you will be jumping rope better than you did when you were a kid. I believe that, as with many things in life, with the right instruction, a positive attitude, and a strong desire, you can do almost anything—yes, even jump rope well.

I am not going to mislead you. It is true that jumping rope is one of the most strenuous activities you can do. But it also burns more calories than almost anything else!

According to Dr. Ken Solis, author of *Ropics: The Next Jump Forward into Fitness*, when jumping rope at a typical rate, which is around 130 jumps per minute (JPM), the body expends the same amount of energy as running nine-to-ten-minute miles or bicycling about thirteen miles per hour. This is extremely demanding for the average inactive person. Even for the athletic person, problems may be encountered. I have experienced firsthand my own tired legs and sore calves from jumping rope.

Fortunately, legs and calves get used to this new activity, and you will not wake up feeling sore every day. If you are inactive and start ANY exercise program, you will be sore. But, jump rope will not make you sore over a long period . . . you just need to get over the hump of not having exercised in a while.

I didn't say that getting in shape was easy, but I did say that jumping rope is absolutely the best, most fun approach. As I will show you, by gradually building your endurance and starting out with very short intervals of jumping interspersed with other exercises, you will quickly get better at it and be surprised at how well you are doing and how well you are feeling.

Real Life Stories About the Jump Rope and How It Changed People's Lives

My client *Susan* is thirty-one years old with a husband, two kids, a house, and a dog. Not only does she not have the time to exercise, but she also truly despises it. (Sound familiar?) Susan insists that she is not coordinated and is certain that her body is no longer capable of changing. The last Cesarean section she had really did her in, and she was very frustrated with her physical well-being.

She came to me looking for the help of a personal trainer. After filling out all the appropriate medical history forms, we followed a friendly workout (very similar to the ones that you will read about in the following chapters). Although most of the workout was walking with only a few thirty to forty-five seconds of interval jumping, Susan was amazed at how much she could do with just a jump rope. She worked her upper body, her lower body, and cardiovascularly, as well.

I have worked with Susan doing many other types of workouts, but jumping became her favorite because she feels that she gets the most out of it—and she finds it the most enjoyable. And, she thought exercise couldn't be *fun*. While she has stuck to her own fitness plan and has stayed motivated enough on her own to stop working with a personal trainer, I do call her up to see how she is doing, and we get together every so often so that she can keep learning new jumps.

Not only has she lost the twelve pounds that were making her feel terrible about herself, but she also learned how important exercise is to enhancing her quality of life. Today, Susan feels better about herself than ever before. She has learned that it is something that she must make time for, or she simply won't feel good. Susan no longer considers herself uncoordinated, and you wouldn't either if you saw her jump rope!

Steve, forty-two, married with two kids, is a successful corporate-account executive in New York City. Along with success came a great deal of business travel. Although Steve had always enjoyed working out and had access to a nearby gym, not all the hotels where he stays on business trips have gym facilities. Steve heard about my jump rope and other workouts through word of mouth and gave me a call.

He already ran on the treadmill, rode an exercise bike, and climbed the StairMaster. He never minded the exercise, he just didn't know what to do when he was traveling or when he was stuck in his apartment on a snowy day. The worst part was working all day, returning to his hotel room, changing for a business dinner, eating and drinking with clients, then heading straight to bed. He said that on these trips, he always felt like a beached whale. He didn't see how he could find a way to exercise during these long and tedious trips.

The jump rope, along with the indoor workouts in this book, Steve believes, saved his life (or, at least added more years to it). I also added variation to Steve's regular gym workouts by showing him how to incorporate the jump rope for intervals in between the exercise machines that he has access to. What he most appreciates about his commitment to fitness—at home and on the road—is that he is setting a great example for his family on how important it is to exercise and stay in shape.

What about the individual who hates going to the gym because they are intimidated by the equipment, the big weightlifting belts, and the massive muscles floating around?

How about people who simply like to exercise by themselves in the privacy of their own homes?

Meet my thirty-eight-year-old client, *Jennifer*, a single woman who disliked going to the gym because it was such a production (going there from work, changing clothing, changing back, and commuting home— the whole evening was gone before she knew it). Jennifer became a "weekend warrior" workout person. During the week, she never had the time to exercise. On the weekends, she'd squeeze in a little cycling or walking. She knew she needed to get into a routine that was more consistent and motivating.

She came to see me, and we worked together for one month, twice a week. We compromised. I encouraged her to continue exercising twice during the week with me and once on the weekend. That way she could do something on her own on Sunday . . . and voilà! she was exercising three times a week. She found this a very doable schedule that didn't interfere much with other things in her life.

I introduced her to the jump rope because she had no cardiovascular machines in her small apartment. She followed the basic warmup (discussed in chapter 4) and then followed workouts very similar to those in the beginner and intermediate chapters of this book. On the third day (on her own, on the weekends), I gave her a choice of doing what she wanted to (Rollerblade, cycle, walk, or follow one of the outdoor workouts).

In just one month, Jennifer seemed to have made exercise a part of her life. She lost five pounds, and her body shape changed. Her buttocks were rounder, her thighs thinner, and her upper body started showing signs of toning up. She mentioned that people at work had noticed her weight loss and that she had more energy. This positive feedback was all Jennifer needed to stay motivated.

Just when she thought it was impossible to fit one more thing in a day, she somehow managed to squeeze exercise into her life. Did you ever hear the saying "Give a busy person something to do, and they will always get it done"? Point made!

Are You Ready to Buy a Jump Rope? Choosing the Proper One

Like buying the right size in-line skates or most comfortable pair of blue jeans, it is important that you choose the appropriate jump rope.

All jump ropes are not created equal—not only in length but in construction, as well. Because the next few paragraphs will be spent discussing the various types of jump ropes on the market, let's talk about one thing that applies to all ropes—the length. A jump rope that is too long for you will not only have too much slack, but will also take more effort to turn (especially if it is "weighted"). Ropes that are too short increase your chance of missing, and they tend to make people

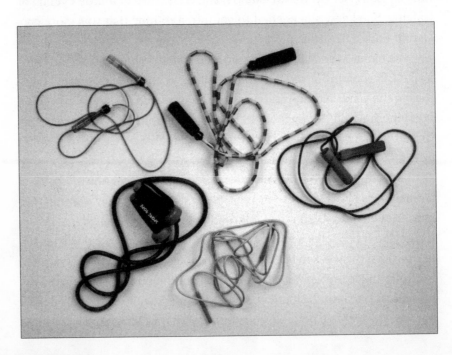

crouch so that the rope doesn't hit their head. This creates poor posture. I could spend a whole chapter on the effects of poor posture on your back and the rest of your body. Simply stated, the proper length of the jump rope is achieved when the end of the handles reaches your armpits while standing on the middle of the rope with one or two feet.

There are many types of ropes available and because this is not an expensive piece of equipment, I recommend that you treat yourself and try a few different styles. The ropes available in stores vary from segmented bead ropes, leather, cotton, and plastic speed ropes, to ropes that are weighted in the handles or in the actual ropes themselves.

Each type of rope has advantages and disadvantages. I do not care for cotton ropes because they feel flimsy. However, they also do not sting as much when you miss a jump. Leather and licorice ropes are fun to jump with when I want to go all out on speed, but when I miss— ouch! Weighted ropes should only be used by the more conditioned individual. Weighted ropes are used to improve upper-body endurance because the arms and shoulders must work hard to keep the rope turning. In my classes we use a rope that is weighted, as opposed to the handles of the rope having weights. Ropes like this have increased work loads because as the rope turns faster, the centrifugal force increases with speed. Don't turn your nose up at a half-pound or one-pound rope. Actually, the centrifugal force (when the rope is whipping around overhead) ends up being equivalent to seven and fifteen pounds respectively because of the momentum of the turns.

I suggest that you go to a good sporting goods store and check out the various ropes. The most important thing is that you feel comfortable holding the rope and jumping with it. There is no right or wrong rope. It is a matter of personal taste.

The Proper Attire for Jumping Rope

As with any sport, it is important that you wear clothing that serves a purpose. I recommend you invest in a good pair of cross-training sneakers. If you have visited a shopping mall recently, you saw how many sports shoes there are. Finding a good shoe should not be a problem. Most of my students and clients wear cross-trainers because these exercises vary greatly each time we work out—which is what these shoes are for. I prefer them for their forefoot cushioning and lateral support.

As for the rest of your body, leotards, shorts, and T-shirts are fine as long as they are breathable and don't inhibit your movement. Of course, depending on your gender, a bra or athletic supporter is crucial.

Headphones are fun to wear and may be securely fastened with holders that can be found in most sporting goods stores. I usually wear a baseball cap which has a dual function—it keeps my hair out of my face and holds my headphones in place.

Comfortable and practical are the two things to keep in mind when you dress for your workout.

CHAPTER 3

TYPES OF JUMPS

Each workout in the following chapters incorporates jumping rope. In this chapter, I will explain to you the specifics of each type of jump—from the most basic to the most advanced. Only you will know when you are ready to go from the basic to the more fancy moves. DON'T RUSH! All these jumps are fun, and I broke each one down into very basic moves. Try them all and have fun. Incorporate more advanced jumps as you go along.

Many factors help to create a varied workout with the jump rope. The combination of the leg movement and cadence at which the jump is performed allows you to adjust the workout from beginner to the most advanced level. For example, take the basic two foot jump. Both feet push off the surface at the same time as the rope turns around. If the focus is on the arms, keep the body more erect and jump and chug the arms faster.

However, if the focus is on the legs, slow the arms down accordingly, but bend into every land almost as if squatting. Note, your heart rate elevates substantially when the range of motion increases in the legs. This is because the lower body carries larger muscles, therefore more blood (O_2) must be pumped into the working muscles to perform the movement.

TIP: Keep in mind that all the following jumps may be made more cardiovascularly demanding if the jump is performed more slowly with a greater range of motion.

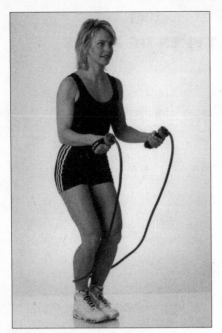

"Ready to jump" position

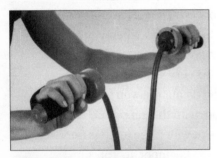

Incorrect form—wrist breaking

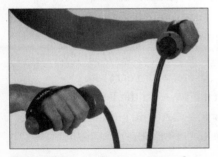

Correct form—wrists are extension of forearms

Arms

There is nothing more hypnotic than watching the rhythmic pace at which a boxer jumps rope. So much attention is given to the foot movement that most people don't give enough credit to how much the arms are working. If the jump rope is weighted, the work load is at least tripled.

Always keep in mind that the speed of the rope comes from the arms, not the feet. The feet simply follow the pace that the arms set. After all, the arms are holding the rope. Since so much time will be spent on footwork in this book, let us set a good foundation for the arms so that their job becomes second nature.

Ready?

Hold the rope in both hands with your rope by your heels in a "ready to jump" position. Your elbows should be slightly bent. Your wrists should be a natural extension of your forearms. Using what I call a "chugging motion," pull your arms toward you, and "flick" the rope overhead. The arms keep chugging back and forth. It is the speed at which you chug that sets the pace of the rope. (Of course, the feet must follow to make the jump successful.)

TIP: BE CAREFUL NOT TO "WRIST BREAK."

Wrist breaking is a term I use with my students and clients not only in jumping rope, but in weightlifting, as well. It is where the wrist rotates around to turn the rope rather than the chugging motion of the arm. Think logically for a moment. Which would have more power behind it, your wrist or your entire arm? Wrist breaking is one of the most common mistakes in jumping rope and can cause injury over time. It may not seem as important in a nonweighted rope because of the ease at which it can be turned. But a weighted rope is another story. Although I have seen professional athletes jumping rope by using the wrists, I do not recommend it because it can cause a great deal of stress on your wrist and hands.

Beginner Jumps

Before you begin practicing the jumps explained below, I want to give you a wonderful (and simple) way to start. Try the jumping patterns first, WITHOUT using a jump rope! Get into the rhythm, the footwork, the feelings, whatever you need to do, before having to worry about turning your arms and swinging a rope over your head. Trust me, it is much easier if you start without the rope!

Okay, here we go.

SINGLE LEG LEAD

One of the basic jumps you might have done as a child was what I call the single leg lead. This is where your dominant leg jumps over the rope first and the trailing leg pushes off. The same movement is repeated. Don't be frustrated if one side is easier to perform than the other. This is quite common. However, do not ignore what you might consider your weaker side. Success breeds success, and it is usually best to try your "weaker side" right away after having successfully completed the jump on the more dominant side.

To change legs, beginners may stop twirling the rope and set themselves up in a "ready to jump" position with their weaker leg ready to lead and the stronger leg ready to trail. Intermediate and advanced jumpers change legs by double bouncing on the dominant leg and kicking forward with the trailing.

TWO FOOT JUMP

The two foot jump is exactly what it says. Start with the rope behind you by your heels in a "ready to

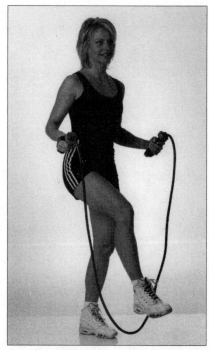

Single leg lead

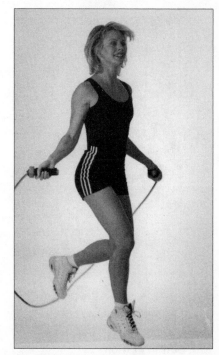

Single leg lead in motion

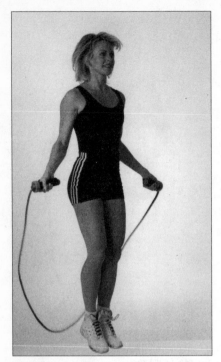

Two foot jump

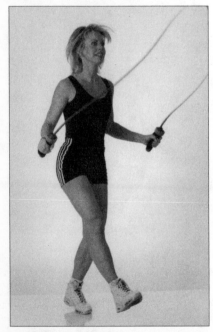

Kick outs in motion

jump" position. Using the chugging motion, bring the rope overhead, and push off with both feet. Bend your knees into each land, readying yourself for the next jump.

When I work with my clients, they seem to find it helpful to say aloud, "JUMP, LAND, JUMP, LAND," and so on. Again, as mentioned in the arms section, if you want to gain speed, it must come from the arms, not the legs. The legs then follow.

KICK OUTS

Kick outs may have been another one of the basic jumps you did as a child. One leg kicks in front while the other leg double-bounces, then the opposite leg kicks in front while the alternate leg double-bounces.

Intermediate Jumps

ALTERNATING FEET
(A.K.A. "JOG PATTERN" OR "BOXERS' JUMP")

Holding the rope in both hands, with the rope behind you by your heels, bring the rope overhead, jumping over it with your leading leg. The trailing leg lifts up over the rope but does not land. Instead, it stays lifted while moving forward to become the leading leg.

I usually tell my students when they are learning this jump to say "RIGHT KNEE, LEFT KNEE, RIGHT KNEE, LEFT KNEE," and so on. It is very common to try to rush the learning process with this jump because we all want to jump rope like a professional boxer. However, I can assure you that even Tyson, Foreman, and Holyfield put many hours into their effortless-looking jumping skills.

Again, the trick is to avoid double bouncing. The speed of the rope is determined by how fast the rope is revolving around. Sound familiar? If it doesn't, please go back, and read the section on arms. As you gain speed with this jump, you will find that the knees will not want to maintain as high a lift. To do this would require a tremendous amount of stamina. Instead, they will naturally lower closer to the floor. You will become very proficient at this jump when your foot is raised only high enough to clear the rope.

JUMPING JACKS

There are two basic steps to the jumping jack pattern. Jump with your feet together, jump with your feet apart. The key is to try to coordinate the jump with turning the rope. Stand in the usual starting position. Bring the rope overhead, and push off with two feet (just like the two foot jump). As your rope comes around for the next revolution, jump over it, but land with your feet apart. You may find it helpful to say "FEET APART, FEET TOGETHER, FEET APART, FEET TOGETHER."

This jump happens to be a terrific example of how one jump can concentrate on various parts of the body. When this jump is performed with speed, the upper and lower body are both working equally hard. However, by slowing the legs and landing in a plié position, this move heavily emphasizes the lower body. It only takes a few of these jumps before your heart rate goes up and your legs burn from the lactic acid buildup. I suggest alternating between these two types of jumps at more advanced levels.

CROSS-COUNTRY SKI JUMP

For most of us, cross-country skiing conjures up an image of long, quiet strides through freshly fallen snow. To watch this sport, it may seem peaceful, serene, and almost effortless. However the leg movements involved engage all the major muscles in the lower body. This makes it one of the most cardio-vascularly challenging sports. The cross-country ski pattern for the jump rope is almost identical to that

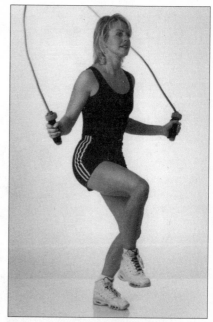

Slow-motion jog pattern—an exaggerated knee lift is helpful in learning jump

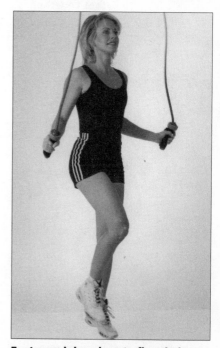

Feet remaining close to floor in jog pattern, as proficiency increases

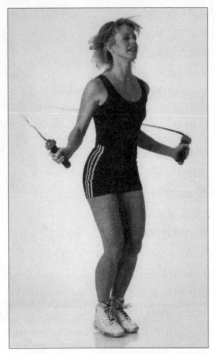

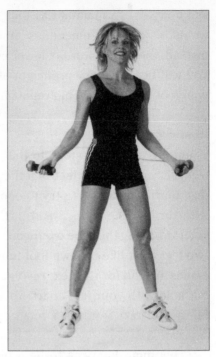

Jumping jack pattern, starting with feet together

Landing with feet apart, toes pointing out, knees bent and over heels

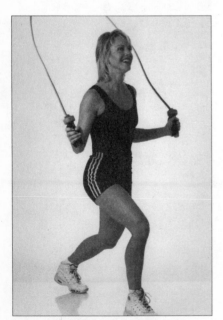

Long stride in performing cross-country ski jump slowly

of the actual sport, with the exception of the height needed to clear the rope while jumping.

In a "ready to jump" position, bring the rope overhead, jump, and after you have cleared the rope, land in the stride position. As the rope comes overhead again, jump in the same stride position but change legs in the air and land with the opposite leg in front. It will help you to say to yourself "CHANGE, CHANGE, CHANGE, CHANGE."

Again the speed of this jump and the length of the strides determine the difficulty of the exercise. Short back-and-forth strides with rapid arm movement is a great overall toner. However, great emphasis may be placed on the legs when the jump is slowed down and the strides become long. Notice again how high the heart rate goes when the legs perform the major muscle moves.

Advanced Jumps

FIGURE EIGHTS

The basic figure eight is an important jump rope pattern to learn. Not only will it serve as a good transitional move when you are feeling fatigued from jumping, but it can also add style to the more accomplished jumper.

To perform the figure eight pattern, simply hold the rope in both hands with the handles together. Keeping the handles together, move your hands and arms in a figure eight (as if the eight is laying on its side). The eight should not exceed the width of your body (the width of your body is usually a pretty good benchmark). The arms are slightly bent, and the power to move the rope around comes from the arms. (Remember, don't use your wrists.) As you gain speed and power, gradually cross one hand over the other while maintaining the same figure eight pattern.

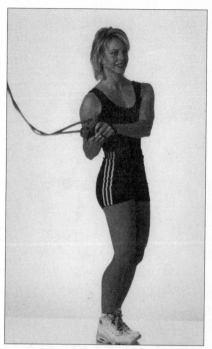

Practicing figure 8s with hands together

TIP: Don't be discouraged if you are still having trouble after the first few times. Chances are you have not jumped rope in a very long time, and this is hard to coordinate. When you get frustrated, stop for a minute, regroup, put things in perspective, and try again. If you get really frustrated, try a jump that you are more successful with, and go back to this one later.

Now that you have established the arm pattern, you begin to add the jump by doing two "eight" patterns with your arms, then uncross your arms and jump in a regular fashion twice. The rhythm is "eight, eight, jump, jump" again "eight, eight, jump, jump." (Arms, arms, jump, jump.)

SKIPPING

Skipping may be broken down into two parts. The first being the two foot jump and the second being a hop.

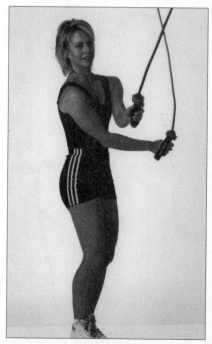

Figure 8s crossing one hand over the other

Start in the "ready to jump" position, and go into the two foot jump. Jump several times like this just to get a rhythm. As you begin to feel more comfortable, lift one knee, and bring the rope around so as to hop over the rope. As the rope comes around again, jump over it using the two foot jump. Continue to bring the rope around again and lift the other knee while hopping over the rope. It will help to say "TWO FEET, ONE FOOT, TWO FEET, ONE FOOT."

The other variation on this jump is to lift your heel back toward your buttocks to work the hamstrings instead of lifting the knee up and working the quadriceps.

CHEST CROSS

Although the level of difficulty is greater, the chest cross pattern is one that everyone likes to master. Not only does this jump look impressive, but most of us who jumped rope as kids probably did it. In my opinion, this is one of the reasons jumping rope is so attractive. There is something to be said for performing an activity as an adult that we did as kids.

TIP: Remember, the patience level required to perform the jump is directly proportional to the difficulty of the jump.

With the above tip in mind, start in the "ready to jump" position and bring the rope overhead using the two foot jump. Because this jump is more complicated, let's break it down into parts.

1) Turn the rope around 3 times using the two foot jump.

2) On the fourth turn, cross one arm over the other so that the elbows are almost aligned on top of each other. Keep in mind that your hands should extend slightly wider than your body.

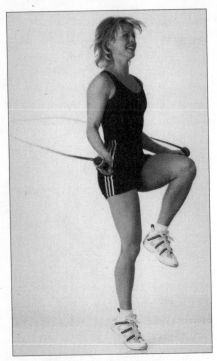

Intentionally lifting knee in skipping pattern

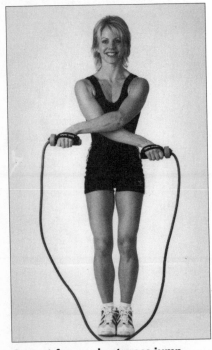

Correct form—chest cross jump

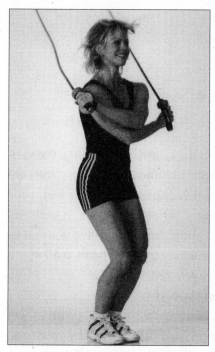

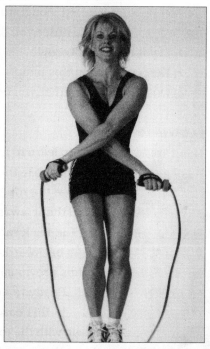

Arms *not* continuing overhead with rope

Cross chest in motion—elbows crossed, hands slightly wider than body

3) Continue to bring the rope overhead, and if you feel so inclined, jump over it as it moves toward your feet. If you feel like you need a transition move, try this: instead of jumping over it on the fourth turn, catch the rope under your toes and hold.

4) Practice this pattern of turning the rope for 3 and crossing on the fourth jump or "catch."

5) Say "one, two, three, cross, one, two, three, cross" as you go along—it'll help.

6) As you begin to successfully clear the rope on the jumps, decrease the 3 jumps and cross to 2 jumps and cross. Hang in there. You are now only one step away from performing this jump.

7) Ready? Jump for one, cross for one, jump for one, cross for one, and so on.

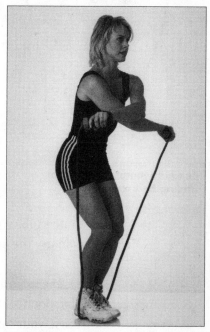

Toe catch

Did you do it? If you did, congratulations. If you didn't, do the following three things in the order you like.

1) Try it again tomorrow.

2) Keep practicing this jump.

3) Do another jump that you can do well.

BACKWARDS JUMP

There are two reasons to learn to jump backwards: 1) to add to the variety of jumps, and 2) to increase the level of difficulty. Because you cannot see the rope as it is approaching your feet, your kinesthetic awareness is heightened when performing the backwards jump. Once you have learned to jump backwards, you may try your hand at all of the jumps previously discussed.

Ready to begin? Good.

In this case, the "ready to jump" position will begin with the rope in front of you down by your toes. Extend your arms in front of you as you lift them up to bring the rope overhead. I have seen beginners perform this jump one of two ways: 1) using the two foot jump, and 2) lifting one foot up at a time. Do what feels most natural to you. It is more important to get a sense of what it feels like to jump backwards.

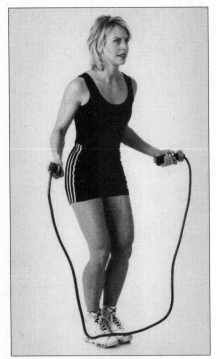

"Ready to jump" position for jumping backwards

TIP: Because people have the tendency to jump too high, or rather overjump, while going backwards, always make sure that you hear the rope hit the ground throughout performing this jump.

TIP: If you have trouble clearing the rope because of the uncertainty of where the rope is and when you should jump, you should use the sound of the rope hitting the ground as a signal to JUMP.

The same rules apply to jumping backwards as jumping forward. Do not double-bounce. Longer slower strides or bending into every land will increase your heart rate. And, the speed of the rope comes from your arms.

The Ultimate Challenge Jumps—
Two Very Advanced Jumps

Believe it or not, in all likelihood, you will master the above jumps and seek new and challenging ones. Or, you just may be the type of person that gets bored easily and wants to live on the edge. Either way, if you are up for it, these next jumps are very advanced. Give them a shot, and have some fun.

BACKWARDS CHEST CROSS

This is a combination of two jumps that I explained earlier. As if the chest cross pattern wasn't hard enough, performing it backwards increases the difficulty level dramatically.

As I did with the other jumps, let me break it down for you. (This one gets complicated, so take each step very slowly.)

1) Stand in a "ready to jump" position for going backwards.

2) Use the two foot jump pattern, and bring the rope overhead to start jumping backwards.

3) As you did with the chest cross forward, jump backwards 3 times, and as the rope comes up from under your feet, cross your arms. Because the rope has some momentum to it, it may actually continue over your head. This is good, and it should give you the confidence to know that you are more than halfway there.

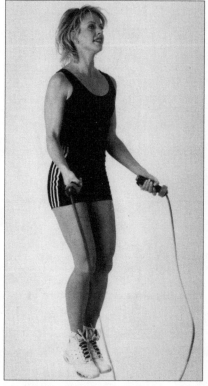

2 foot starting position for jumping backwards

TIP: There are a couple of tips to keep in mind here that will help make the jump successful. There is a tendency to bring the hands up overhead to help the rope over—DON'T! The arms stay crossed at the chest as a unit. A slight lift from the arms will help the rope go around. The other common mistake people tend to make is that they start to hunch over because they are afraid the rope won't make it around. Keep your body erect! It will give the arms more power because the leverage is better.

4) After you have successfully crossed your arms, jumped backwards, and cleared the rope, it is time to uncross the rope so that you are jumping backwards again. It is best to go back into the pattern of jumping with the initial pattern of jumping three times backwards and then crossing the rope again until you feel you develop a nice rhythm.

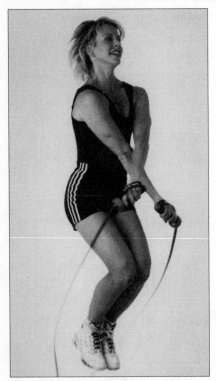

It is best to say aloud, "jump, two, three, cross, jump, two, three, cross."

5) Now you are ready to do singles. Take out the second and third backwards jump and say aloud (of course you want your body to respond), "jump one, cross one, jump one, cross one."

How did you do? Whether you were successful in clearing the rope is not important. It is more important that you tried. Furthermore, the fact that you were even ready for this jump is an accomplishment.

Crossing arms on second turn of rope

BACKWARDS JUMPING JACKS

Again you are combining two jumps. I'm sure by now you can see that all of the jumps that were discussed previously may be performed backwards. Some are harder to do than others.

Here we go.

1) In a "ready to jump" backwards position, bring the rope overhead, and start jumping backwards using the two foot jump.

2) Start turning the rope at a fairly slow speed, and land on both feet.

3) When you feel comfortable, land with your feet apart instead of together.

4) To perform the jump successfully, the feet land either apart or together with every turn of the rope.

5) Say aloud, "feet apart, feet together, feet apart, feet together."

TIP: Remember to start slowly. Speed will come when you are more comfortable with the jump. This holds true for all the jumps discussed in this chapter.

These represent a wide variety of jumps from the basic to the very complicated and advanced. It doesn't matter which ones you master and which ones you choose to avoid. What matters is that you try what feels comfortable and that you get moving and jumping!

Please remember to flip back to this chapter often. You will especially need to refer to these jumps before and during each of your workouts so that you: 1) choose a jump to use during the workout; 2) remind yourself of the proper, safe steps and instructions for that jump; and 3) push yourself a little bit more by trying one other jump if you feel ready.

Get on your workout clothes, and get ready to warm up for jumping!

CHAPTER 4

GETTING STARTED:
THE WARMUPS AND THE COOLDOWNS

The most important element of any exercise program is proper preparation.

The purpose of the warmup is to prepare your body for the demands of aerobics and calisthenics. This is done by raising your internal body temperature. As your body temperature increases, more blood flows to the working muscles and more oxygen is released. The goal of the warmup should be to raise your body temperature approximately four degrees so that you sweat.

Some of the physiological benefits of the warmup include a higher metabolic rate, increased blood flow to the muscles, higher rate of exchange between blood and muscles, more oxygen released within muscles, increased muscle elasticity, increased flexibility of tendons and ligaments, and a rehearsal effect. The rehearsal effect allows the body to practice some of the muscular patterns that are used later in the workout.

The warmup I describe in this book will take approximately five minutes. The muscle joint preparation and stretching should be done at the beginning and end of EVERY workout. The muscle joint preparation in the warmup allows the muscles to be stretched further during the activity so that damage and injury does not occur.

The primary function of the cooldown is to lower your heart rate from a cardiovascular workout, as well as to stretch the muscles again to enhance flexibility. Flexibility is important in preventing injury as well as improving performance. By stretching the muscles while they are warm, there is less chance of tissue damage. There is also an increase in the amount of elongation that remains after the stretch is removed. The control and speed at which the stretch is performed is VERY important. Ballistic or "bouncy type" stretches should be avoided because they can cause injury.

The Warmup!

The movements in the following warm-up routine will specifically prepare your body for jumping rope and all the interval circuit training workouts in this book. As you follow this portion, it not only ensures that your appropriate muscles are saturated with blood so that they can perform the movements with greater ease, but it also provides a rehearsal effect. This means that your body has a chance to practice the patterns similar to those used in the rest of the workout. For example, warm-up exercises like "push-releases" will be used to prepare your calves, ankles, and feet for jumping and landing. The warmup will also include some full-body movements to incorporate more muscle groups and, therefore, raise your body temperature. A series of muscle joint preparation exercises will also be included in this section to prepare your body for these full-range movements at a more vigorous pace.

The following warmup may be used for all the workouts in this book. This may be performed indoors or outdoors.

Here we go.

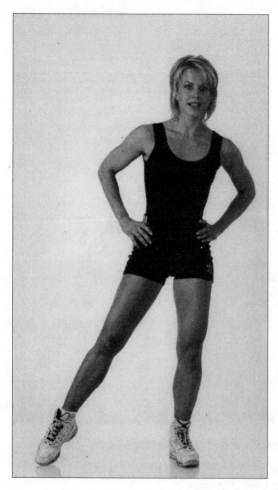

1) Start by alternating toe taps on the floor. Tap right. Tap left. Repeat for 8 counts.

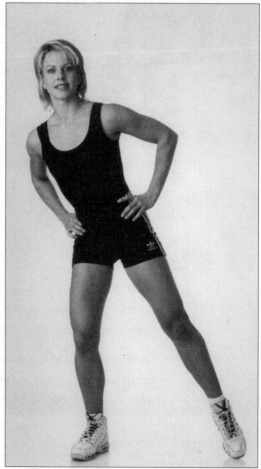

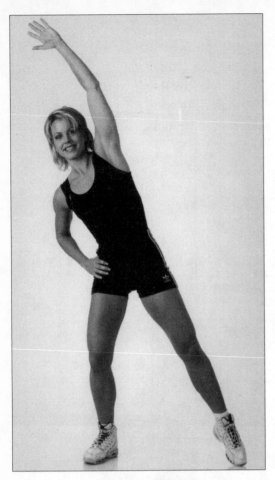 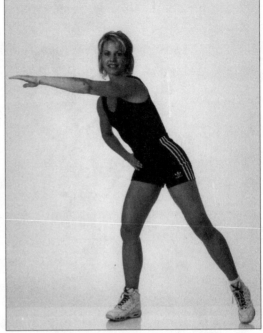

2) While still tapping on the floor with alternating feet, reach your arms up overhead one at a time as you are stretching from side to side. Repeat this movement for 8 counts.

3) While continuing to tap your feet from side to side, bring your arms in front of you one at a time, reaching from side to side. Repeat this movement for 8 counts.

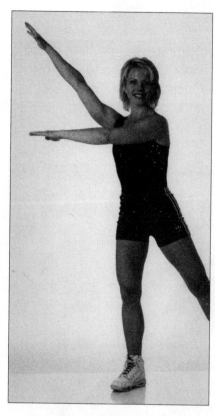

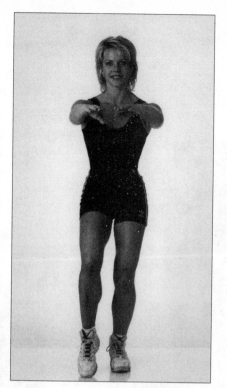

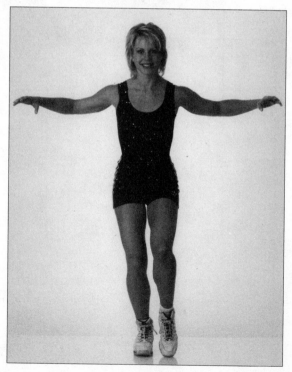

4) Swing both arms from side to side while tapping your feet. Repeat for 8 counts.

5) Step and touch from side to side, while the arms pull back and out to your sides, parallel to your shoulders. Repeat 4 times.

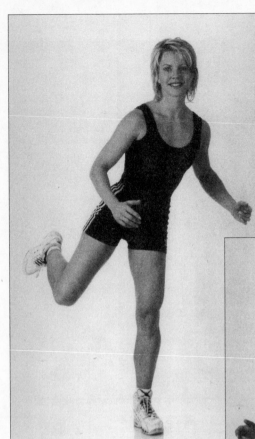

6) Alternate lifting your heel back toward your buttocks 8 times. Then do doubles (lifting two times on each side).

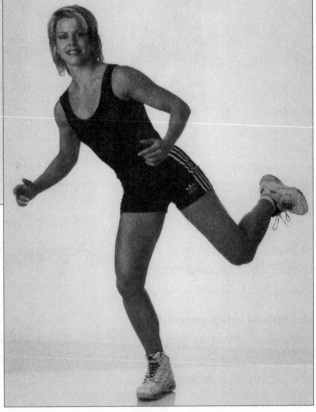

7) Step and touch again from side to side with your hands on your hips. Repeat 4 times.

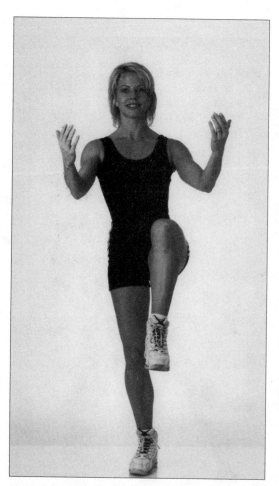 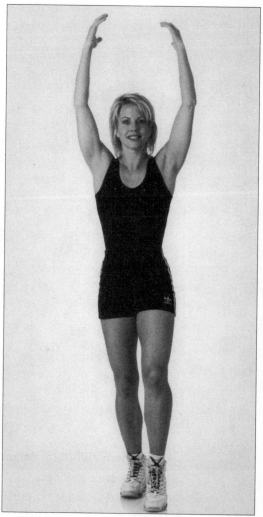

8) Alternate lifting your knees up while your arms pull out and down from over your head to your shoulders. Repeat for 8 counts. Then do doubles (lifting two times on each side).

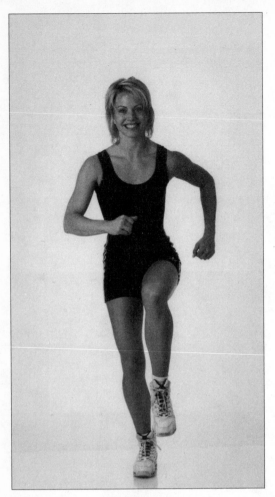

9) March it out in place for 8 counts. Then spread your feet wider apart, and march in place for 8 counts. Bring your feet back together, and repeat the series 2 more times.

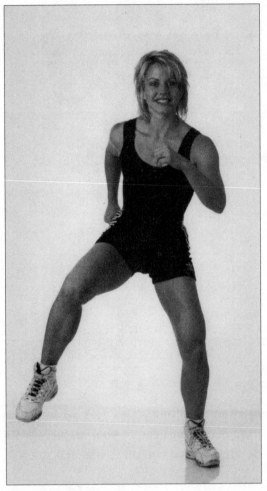

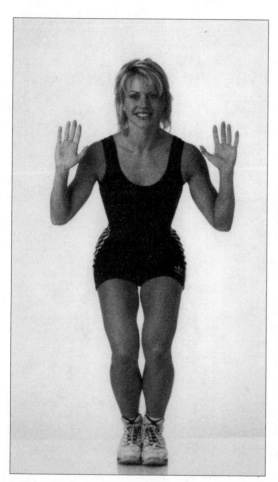
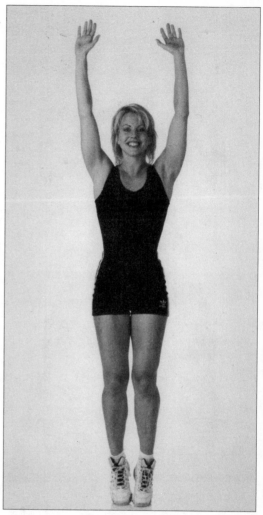

10) With your feet together, perform 8 push-releases while simultaneously pushing your arms up in the air. The push-release begins with the weight of the body forward, supported mostly by the front part of the foot (or ball of the foot). Then, you should forcefully push away from the floor while pointing the toe, so that the foot raises slightly off the floor. Then lower yourself to the floor while bending your knees.

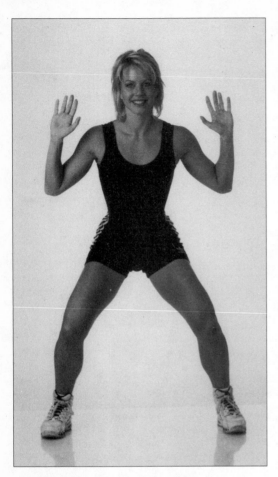 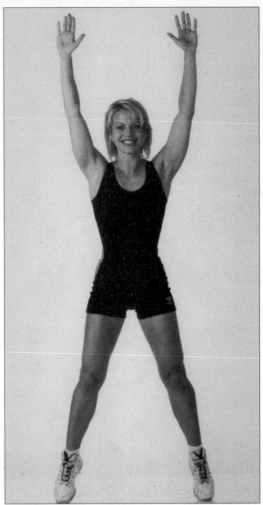

11) Repeat movement number 10 with feet wide apart for 8 counts.

12) Now for the muscle joint preparation portion of the warmup. This is a good place for you to start using your rope as a stretching tool. When you do these stretches, instead of just using your hands to pull, reach, and stretch, you can fold your rope in half or quarters and hold your foot with it.

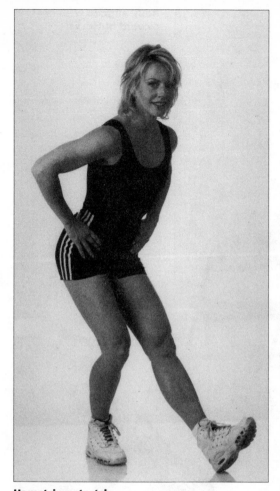

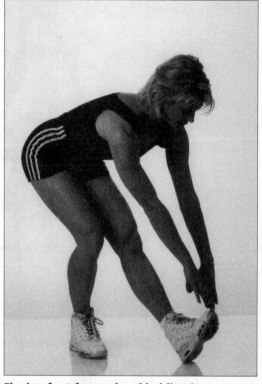

Hamstring stretch

Flexing foot forward and holding it, for greater stretch

For your hamstrings, start by bringing your right foot in front and digging your heel into the floor. Take a deep breath while bringing your arms up over your head and reaching them down toward your toe. Keep your heel anchored into the floor, and pull your buttock away so the muscle lengthens. Repeat on the other side. (For a variation, you can use the rope folded in quarters placed under your foot and in each hand to reach for the stretch.)

TIP: If you are indoors this may also be done by placing your foot on any steps in your home. If you are outside, you may use the curb.

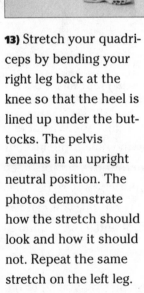

**Body aligned with heel
toward buttocks**

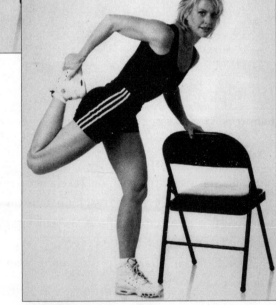

13) Stretch your quadriceps by bending your
right leg back at the
knee so that the heel is
lined up under the but-
tocks. The pelvis
remains in an upright
neutral position. The
photos demonstrate
how the stretch should
look and how it should
not. Repeat the same
stretch on the left leg.

Incorrect form

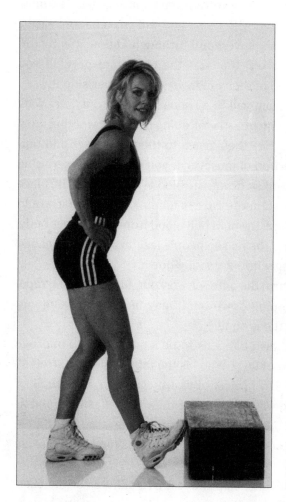

14) To stretch the calves, flex your right foot toward you, and place it heel down against a wall, a step, or if you're outside, you may use the curb. Keep this leg straight without locking your knee, and lean forward so that most of the weight is on the heel. Repeat on the other foot.

How did you do? You should feel warmed up and ready to exercise. Please remember to take your time during the warmup, and do not cut any corners. If you try to rush through it, you will not be preparing your body properly, and you might get injured when you exercise.

The Cooldown!

The cooldown is done after you have completed one of the jump rope workouts in this book. The purpose of the cooldown at the end of the workout is to lower your heart rate and stretch your muscles. The muscles at this point are saturated with blood and will stretch more easily.

Do not skip this part of the workout. Although I know it is tempting to say, "I did the exercises, that was the important part," if you understand the importance of the cooldown, you'll never skip it.

Did you ever hear a coach yell to a runner, "Walk it out," or "Walk it off"? There is a very specific reason for doing this. The working muscles require blood that carries the oxygen to them. The legs and buttocks have the largest portion of muscles. If you have been exercising vigorously and then stop and sit down, the blood (O_2) goes to the place where it is needed the most. In the case of a human being, that would be our lower body. Therefore, it would pull blood from your upper body, including your head. This is the reason people feel dizzy or lightheaded if they just stop exercising without cooling down.

So, please do not perform the outdoor workout, finish jumping rope, and find a park bench to plop down on. It may be the last thing you remember before hitting the ground.

The cooldown period also happens to be a great time to improve flexibility. Think of a piece of taffy. When is the taffy easiest to stretch? When it is cold or warm? The answer obviously is warm. Well, think of your muscles in the same way. They are at their most flexible point at the end of the workout. Your body temperature is elevated. Your muscles are saturated with blood. Take advantage of this time to gain some flexibility.

If you are pressed for time, skip the last five minutes of the exercise part and do the cooldown. Your body will love you for it. Stretching prevents injury in many areas including but not limited to the lower back, hamstrings, calves, shoulders, and quadriceps. It also feels great.

Ready to Cool Down?

1) If you are outside, walk around for 2–3 minutes (around your house, around the block, wherever). If you are indoors, walk in place or around your home for 2–3 minutes. Keep walking if your heart rate has not come down yet. Do this until you feel like you can breathe normally.

2) Now for the stretching part (in the cooldown, your flexibility will increase from the warmup). Stand up straight near a wall (or a tree, if outdoors), feet parallel about one foot from the wall. Stretch upward

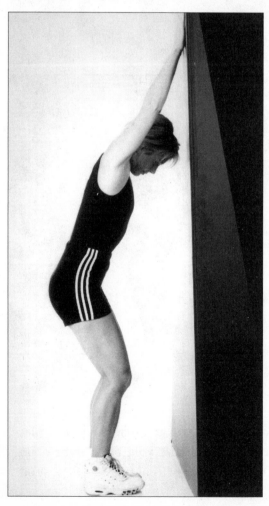

with your entire body using your fingertips— don't let your elbows touch the wall. Let your fingers "walk" up the wall or tree as far up as they will go, and use this to pull your body up for a stretch. Hold for 10–15 seconds.

3) Now stand back up, and stretch your calves. Flex your right foot toward you, and place it heel down, against a wall, a step, or if you are outdoors, the curb. Keep the right leg straight without locking your knee, and lean forward so that most of your weight is on that heel. Repeat on the other side.

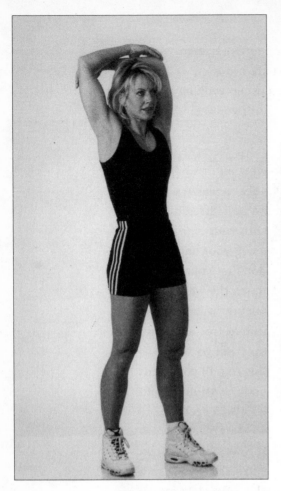

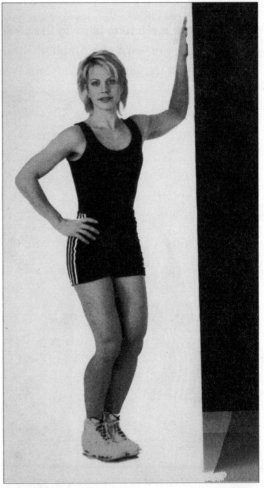

4) Stretch your triceps by bending your elbow up over your head. Stretch and reach up and over with your elbow. Hold this stretch for 10–15 seconds.

5) Stretch your chest by bending your arm at a right angle, and place it against the corner of a wall (or tree). Turn your body in the opposite direction. You should be turning away from the wall. Repeat on the other side.

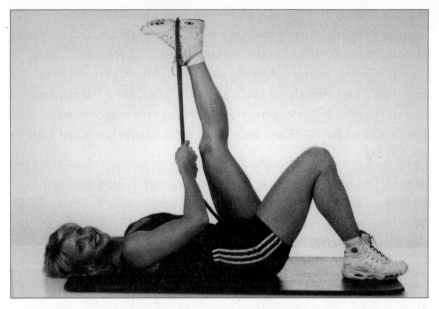

Start of stretch

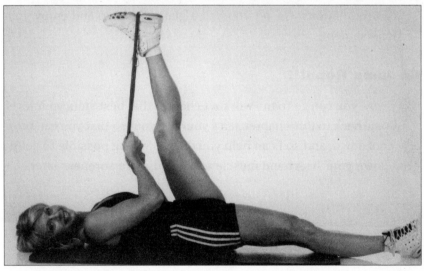

Lowering leg to floor, if able to stretch more

6) Now for the floor stretches. Lie down on the floor (with or without a mat) with your knees bent. Place the rope around the arch of your right foot, and gently stretch and extend your right leg up. Hold for 10–15 seconds. The goal of this stretch is for your leg to be as perpendicular to the floor as possible. Don't worry if you cannot get it straight up. On the other hand, if you are able to bring your leg completely perpendicular and it still doesn't feel like a challenge, then unbend your other leg, and lay it flat on the floor.

7) Before doing the previous stretch on your other side, remain in the same position as above (with your right leg upright), and do the next stretch. Holding the rope (still around the arch of your foot), drop your leg gently up and out to the side of your body (toward your hip)—hold and stretch for 10–15 seconds. Then, for a full range of motion, stretch to the opposite side (almost crossing over your left leg/hip). Hold for 10–15 seconds. Now, repeat stretches 6 and 7 on the left leg.

8) Next, lie on your stomach, legs and body flat. Bend your right leg so that your heel is touching or almost touching your buttocks. Hold 10–15 seconds. Now do the other leg.

You have completed all the stretches, and you should feel completely stretched, cooled down, and extremely proud of yourself!

Congratulations! Go get yourself a glass of water, and enjoy your accomplishment!

Go Jump Rope!!!

Okay, now you can go to the workout chapter that best suits your level.

Come back to this chapter AFTER your workout so that you can properly cool down, and so I can help you do everything possible to gently calm down your heart and muscle and avoid extra soreness later.

CHAPTER 5

JUMP ROPE FOR THE BEGINNER

The following three workouts were created for the person just starting out. This includes individuals who have recently embarked on an exercise program; those who have exercised for a period of time, but who have never jumped rope before, and/or done strength-training exercises; and, those who have not exercised in a very long time (no matter how athletic you were as a child or teenager).

All the workouts in this chapter take no longer than fifteen to twenty minutes to complete. Keep in mind that these workouts are VERY flexible. There are many, many ways for you to vary them. You may feel that you can jump longer than the fifteen to thirty seconds that I put in the workout. If you can go longer, do it! On the other hand, you may have a difficult time clearing the rope, coordinating the jumps, or jumping for more than a couple of seconds. That's okay, too! You can still do the workout (no excuses).

If you cannot clear the rope, try this: hold the rope in one hand, and turn the rope around. This way you may practice jumping in time with the rope without the worry and frustration of missing it . (If you use this technique, remember to change hands.) I promise you, you will get better and better at it.

There may be days when you have extra time, but you are not yet at the intermediate level. If that is the case, you should try to increase

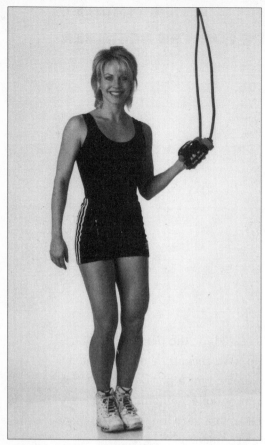

Holding rope ends in one hand, turning rope, and practicing jumping in time

your workout time by fast-walking longer in between the steps that I have laid out for you. If you begin to master the basic jumps, but are not ready for the intermediate workout, then you should do the beginner workouts, but start to challenge yourself by expanding your jumping repertoire. Longer, shorter walking, more or fewer jumps, different jumps—the more you vary, the less bored and frustrated you are likely to get.

YOU ARE TRULY THE MASTER OF YOUR WORKOUT.

You will know when you are ready for the next level (the intermediate workouts in the next chapter) when you feel you've not only mastered these workouts in terms of the jumping skills, but more importantly, when you feel you are performing the workouts with greater ease. For example, where your legs may have had that burning sensation on the twelfth lunge when you started out, they don't anymore. Or, you may have been jumping for thirty to forty-five seconds and was sure there was no way that you could do one more jump, but now you feel you could definitely go longer. Your balance will also improve and, therefore, you may want to add an arm exercise while you do the leg exercises, rather than holding on to something for balance.

I have found—and I know that my clients agree—that one of the most interesting things about incorporating a good exercise program into your life is that you become extremely in touch with your body. In the same way that your body may say, "My legs are burning, and I have to stop," it can also say, "This feels like it is getting easier, and I don't feel the same burning I did a couple of weeks ago."

It may be a cliché, but it is true. Today is the first day of the rest of your life. It is up to you to make it a healthier life. So pick up a jump rope, set twenty minutes aside, take a deep breath, and start getting healthy!

Indoor Workout # 1 for Beginners

First, read through this section to see what you need, and assemble the items near you so you won't have to interrupt your workout.

1) Follow the warmup in chapter 4.

2) Perform 8–12 squats, keeping your knees over your toes and pushing your buttocks back, as if you are about to sit down. Lower your body to where your knee is at a right angle. Use anything you need to help you keep your balance and keep the correct form. Hold a doorknob, railing, banister, or the back of a chair, and start squatting! Make the squats slow and even.

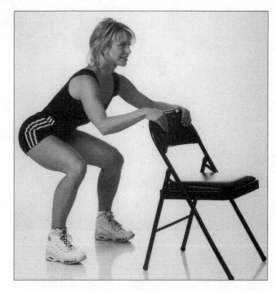

3) Unfold your rope, and jump rope (remember, any jumping style discussed in chapter 3 is fine—just take it easy!) for 15–30 seconds.

4) Now, step from side to side to bring your heart rate down enough to do the next move.

5) Stand with your feet shoulder-width apart. Face a wall, and place your hands against the wall at chest level and as wide or slightly wider than your body. Bend your elbows so that your body is closer to the wall, and then straighten your arms (without locking your elbows) to push your body away. These are a type of push-up and will help to strengthen your arms. Repeat this 16 times at an even pace.

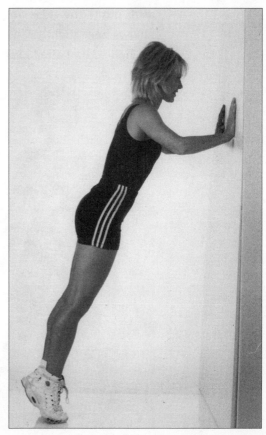

TIP: Remember that movements should not be done quickly, or you will end up using momentum, not muscle, to complete the exercise.

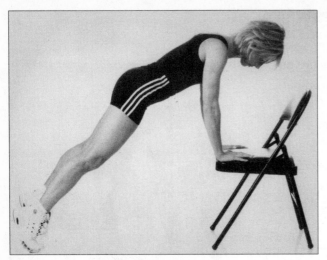

TIP: If you feel that this type of push-up is not much of a challenge for you, then try using the back of a couch or something that is lower to the floor—but will not move. You may also perform them on the floor. Get on your hands and knees so that your hands are in line with your chest. Lower your body toward the floor, and straighten your arms back out again.

6) Holding a can or bottle in each hand (same exact weight in each hand)—or using 3- to 5-pound free weights—stand with your feet apart, knees slightly bent, and your hands by your side. Raise your arms out to the sides no higher than your shoulders, keeping your elbows bent slightly. The weights in your hands should be heavy enough so that after 12–16 repetitions, you are fatigued.

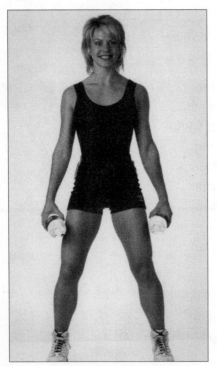

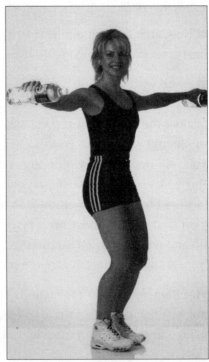

7) Pick up your rope, and jump using one of the beginner jumps for 15–30 seconds.

8) Walk around, or step side to side, to bring your heart rate down.

9) Holding on to a chair, couch, or railing, stand with your feet together. Perform lunging backwards by extending your right leg behind you so that your front knee goes no lower than a 90-degree angle. Keeping the weight on your left leg, push your heel into the floor enough to bring your right leg back to standing position. Repeat the lunge 8–12 times.

10) Repeat on the other side.

11) Pick up the jump rope, and jump for 15–30 seconds.

12) Step from side to side, and follow the cooldown in chapter 4.

CONGRATULATIONS! You have completed your first workout! How do you feel? Was the workout very, very hard? Or was it easier than you thought it would be? You should constantly evaluate your progress so that you know when to move on to a harder workout.

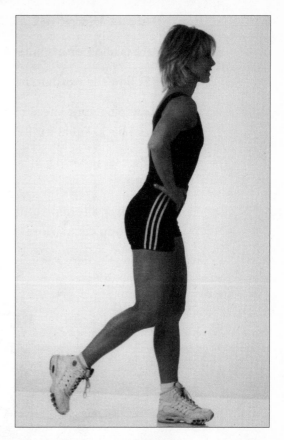

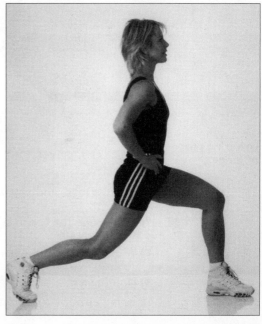

Indoor Workout #2 for Beginners

Here is another beginner workout for you to try.

1) Follow the warmup in chapter 4.

2) Keeping your knees over your toes, and pushing/sitting your buttocks back, squat for 8–12 reps.

3) Pick up the rope, and jump for 15–30 seconds using any one of the jumps.

4) Walk or alternate lifting your knees until your heart rate drops to where you can perform the next move.

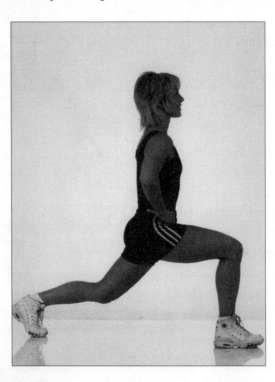

Lowering phase of lunge

5) Perform 8–12 forward lunges on your right leg. Start with your feet together, and step forward with your right leg. Lower your body to where your front knee goes no lower than a right angle. Push back off with your right leg so that you are in a standing position again. (Remember, you may hold on to anything that helps you to keep your balance.)

6) Change legs, and repeat the exercise on the left side.

7) Jump rope for 15–30 seconds using any jump.

8) Walk for a minute or so, and catch your breath for the next move.

9) Holding a can or bottle in each hand (same weight in each hand)—or using either 3- or 5-pound free weights—stand with your feet apart and your hands by your sides. Raise your arms out to the sides no higher than your shoulders, keeping your elbows bent slightly. The weights in your hands should be heavy enough so that after 12–16 repetitions, you are fatigued.

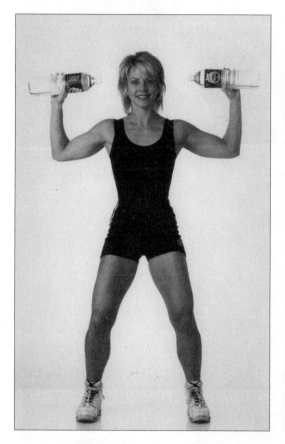 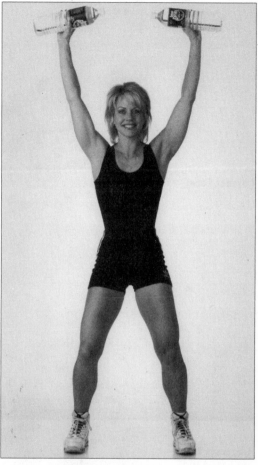

10) Keep your weights in your hands, bend your elbows, and bring your hands up to your shoulders with your palms facing forward. Push the weights up over your head keeping them in line with your shoulders. Lower them back to shoulder height, and repeat the exercise 12–16 times.

11) Jump rope for 15–30 seconds.

12) Walk until your heart rate comes down so that your breathing becomes more regular.

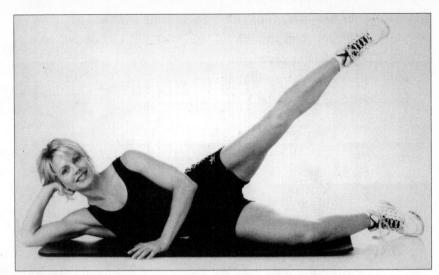

Correct form

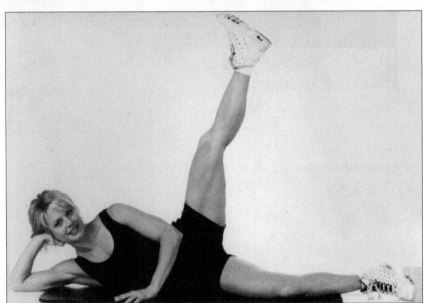

**Incorrect form—
leg lifted too
high and knee
rotated upward**

13) Perform side leg lifts by lying on your side with your knees
slightly bent. Keep your foot angled downward. Lift and lower your
leg at a slow and even pace. Be careful not to turn your knee up
toward the ceiling. Repeat 12–16 lifts.

14) Change legs, and repeat on the other side.

15) Ready to cool down? Follow the cooldown in chapter 4.

Outdoor Workout For Beginners

1) Follow the warmup.

2) Start to walk outside at a moderate pace. While walking, fold the rope into quarters, and placing one end in each hand, pulling the rope taut, extend your arms up, and push the rope overhead—up and down in front of you to chest level. Repeat 8 times.

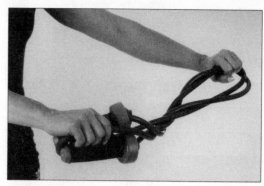

Rope in quarters

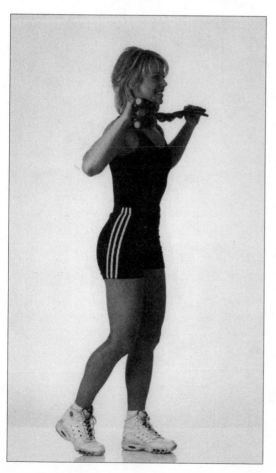

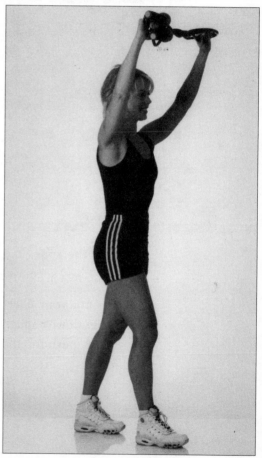

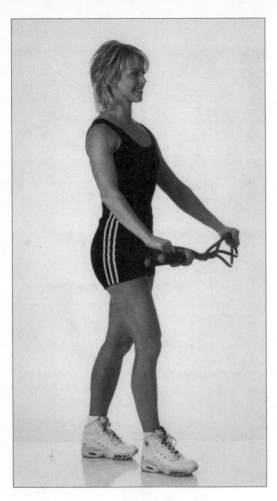

3) Keep walking, and bring the rope in front of you with your arms extended straight out without locking your elbows. Lift as high as your forehead, and lower to the front of your body. Keeping the rope taut, repeat 8 times.

4) Unfold the rope, and jump for 15–30 seconds.

5) Walk until your heart rate comes down enough for you to perform the next move.

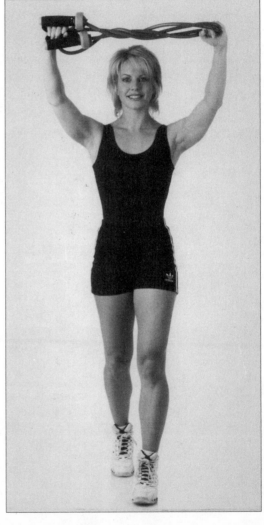

6) Keeping your knees over your toes and sitting your buttocks back, perform 8–12 full-range squats. If you need to hold on to something for balance, find a park bench, and put the rope down to hold on, or, use the rope by placing it around a street sign or tree. Then, hold on to the rope part itself, not the handles, and, keeping the rope taut, sit back into your squat position. (Your heart rate may go up when you do squats. If that happens, you should walk after the squats until you feel that you are ready to jump again.)

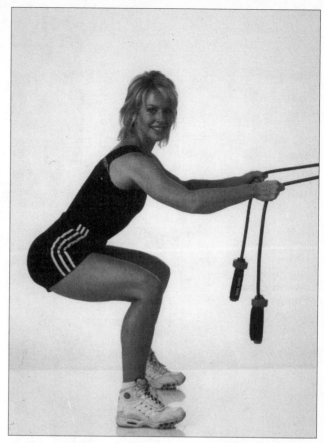

Rope around tree or street sign for squats

7) Unfold the rope, and jump for 15–30 seconds.

8) Again, you may hold on for balance. Stand in a lunge position. Your right leg should be forward with your knee aligned over your toes, and your left leg is back on the ball of your foot. Hold on for balance with your right hand, and place the folded rope in your left hand. In the lunge, the weight of your body is always on the front leg. Now, lower your body to where your knee is at a right angle, and then rise back to your starting lunge position. Perform 8–12 lunges.

TIP: If your balance is good, you may want to place your foot on a curb.

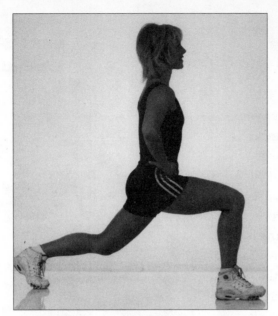

Lowering phase of lunge

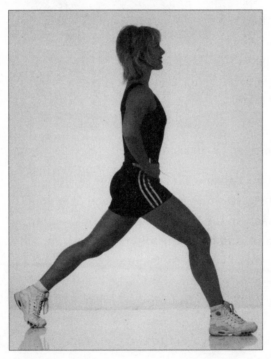

Rising phase of lunge

9) Repeat the same lunges on the other side. This time the left leg is forward, hold on with your left hand, and place the rope in your right hand.

10) Pick up the rope, and jump for 15–30 seconds.

11) Walk it out, and bring your heart rate down.

12) Stay outdoors, or go inside for the cooldown (chapter 4).

How did you do?

These three beginner variations should keep you challenged and busy for a while. They should also help you to realize that you can make a difference in your body and in your life by doing rather simple, but effective and fun, workouts.

Stick with it, and I promise you that in a matter of weeks, you will be turning the page and going on to the intermediate jumps.

Be proud of yourself! You have taken the first step.

CHAPTER 6

THE NEXT STEP:
JUMP ROPE FOR THE INTERMEDIATE

First of all, let me congratulate you for making it to this point.

By now, you should be feeling more comfortable with the jump rope, and although you may not have perfected the first jumps, you should be doing them with greater ease and be excited about learning some new ones to add to your repertoire.

All the workouts in this section can be accomplished in thirty minutes. Keep in mind that you may do intermediate jumps in all the jump sections, or you may do beginner jumps in those sections.

You may not need to "walk it out" to get your heart rate down during some of these steps. If that is the case, omit it, and go right to the next step.

Use your creativity, and design your own workout—add extra seconds to the jumping, change your jumps. These workouts are designed to get you up and moving and help you to progress. Also, you should keep in mind that all these workouts can be done with a friend—double the fun and double the motivation! (For more ways you and your partner can work together, see chapter 9.)

The jump rope portions in these intermediate workouts are slightly longer than in the beginner sections. As an intermediate, you will now start to use your arms and legs together, which will further your coordination and balance capabilities.

There are also some lunges in the intermediate workouts that are not average lunge forward or lunge back-type moves. Take the time to read through the workouts the night before or maybe practice the moves in the mirror so you do not feel like you are breaking the flow of your workout.

Good Luck!

Indoor Workout #1 for Intermediates

1) Follow the warmup.

2) Unfold the rope, and use one of the beginner jumps to jump for 30–45 seconds.

TIP: If you choose single leg leads, make sure you don't always lead with the same leg. You want to develop both sides of your body equally.

3) Walk for 1 minute around your house or apartment (or go on to step 4 if you feel that your heart rate is down).

4) Standing with your feet together, squat to your right side by leading with your right leg. Bring your feet back together, and then squat to your left side. This counts as one repetition. Perform 8 of them.

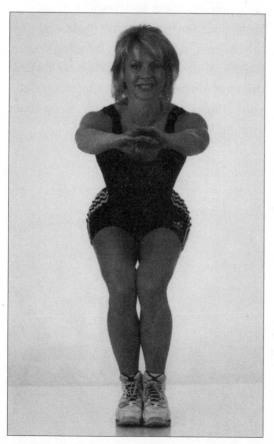 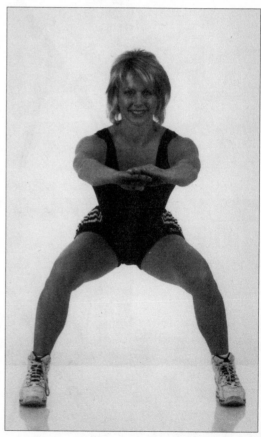

5) Pick up weights, cans, or bottles heavy enough to fatigue you after 12–16 repetitions. Stand with your feet shoulder-width apart, and perform lateral raises by holding the weights by your side and raising your arms out to the side no higher than your shoulders, and then lower them back to your sides.

6) Pick up your jump rope, and do one of the intermediate jumps. Jump for 30–45 seconds.

Starting position

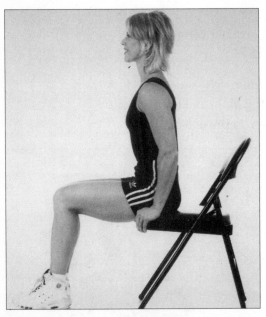

7) Walk for 1 minute to lower your heart rate (or move on to step 8).

8) Triceps dips: Sit on the edge of a folding, kitchen, or living-room chair. With your palms facing down and your fingertips wrapped around the end of the chair, your hands should be hip-width apart. Move your buttocks off the chair, and lower them to the floor by bending your elbows. Your elbows should go no lower than a 90-degree angle. Be sure not to let your elbows go out to the side. Keep them straight back. Do 8–12 reps.

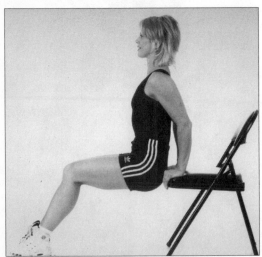

Preparing for the lowering phase

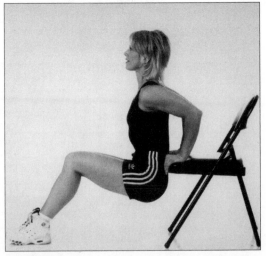

Lowering phase—elbows no lower than 90 degrees

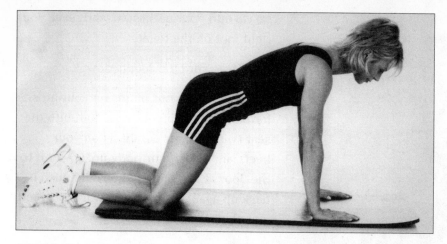

Starting position for push-up

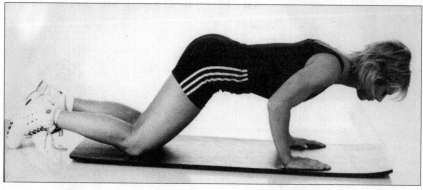

Lowering position for push-up

9) Perform push-ups on your hands and knees (you may want to fold up a towel and put it beneath your knees). Your hands should be level with your chest and about as wide or slightly wider than your body. Lower your upper body to the floor so that your elbows make a right angle, and then push up by straightening your arms without locking your elbows. Repeat 12–16 times.

10) Pick up your rope, and do one of the intermediate jumps. You may even try challenging yourself by trying to jump longer. Combine one of the intermediate jumps with a beginner jump, if you need to. For example, do the jumping jack pattern for 30 seconds, a single leg lead for 15 seconds, and then switch to the other leg for 15 seconds. Guess what? You just did a minute!

11) Walk it out for a minute so that your heart rate has a chance to come down.

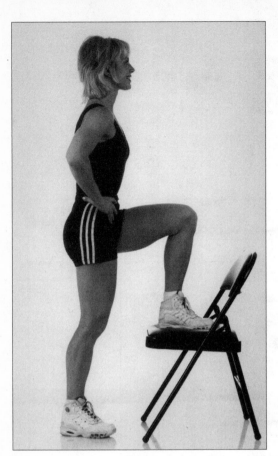

12) Go into your bathroom, and place your right foot on the toilet.

TIP: Make sure the seat is down!

You may place your hands on your hips for balance. Push your right foot into the seat (with greater emphasis on your heel), and push your body up. Lower it to the floor at the same tempo, and push it back up again. Your left leg will lift behind you. Repeat 12–16 times.

13) Change legs, and repeat on the other side.

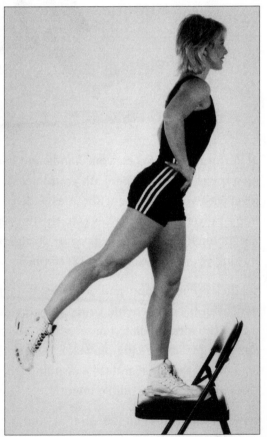

14) If you want to finish with a bang, jump rope one last time for 30–45 seconds. Or maybe you can do a minute?

15) Follow step 1 in the cooldown, then go to the next step here.

16) Lower your body to the floor with your legs lengthened out and your feet turned out to the side. Place your hands behind your head. Keeping your head in line with your spine, neck relaxed, contract your abdominal muscles, and lift your upper body. (Remember that your back should be flat and you are tilting your pelvis.) Keeping the contraction on your abdominals, lower your body to the floor without resting, and raise it back up again. Do 16 of these full-range abdominal exercises, and then pulse 16 times.

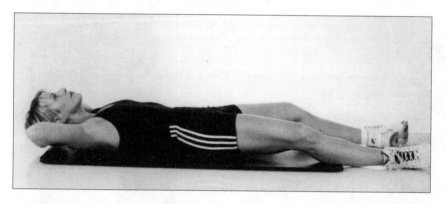

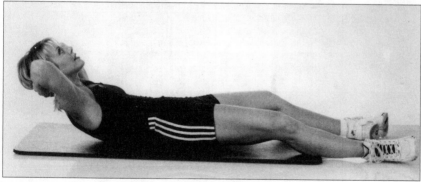

17) Finish the cooldown, starting with step 2.

Indoor Workout # 2 for Intermediates

1) Follow the warmup.

2) Stand with your feet slightly wider than shoulder-width apart. Fold the rope in half. Hold the rope overhead using a wide grip in each hand. As you lower your body into the squat position (buttocks drop no lower than your knees), pulse for three counts before you rise. Your arms will simultaneously pull down from overhead toward your chest. Pulse for three counts, and push back up. Repeat 8–12 times.

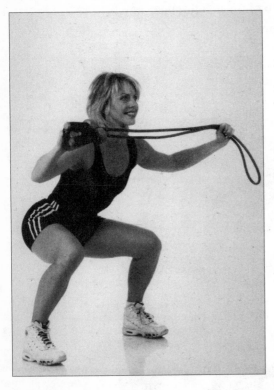

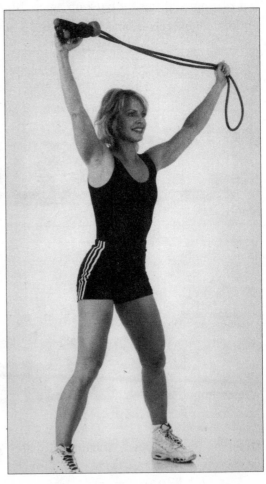

3) Unfold the rope, and using one of the beginner jumps, jump for 30–45 seconds.

4) Walk for 1 minute to lower your heart rate, or you may move on to step 5.

5) Perform 12–16 triceps dips using a folding chair, kitchen chair, or the end of a couch.

6) You may hold on to a chair for this next set of lunges. Fold your rope into eighths or use a can or bottle for weights. Now, stand with your right leg forward in a lunge position. The chair should be on your right side. Hold the weight in your left hand. As you lower your body on the lunge, raise your arm out to the side. As you rise from the lunge, lower your arm to your side. Repeat 8–12 times.

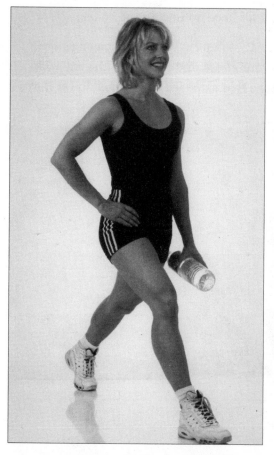

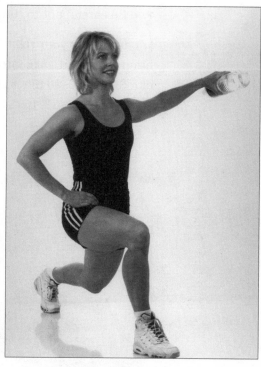

7) Ready for the other side? Change legs (the chair is now on your left side, and your left leg is forward). Hold the weight in your right hand. Repeat 8–12 times.

8) Unfold the rope, and jump for 30–45 seconds using one of the intermediate jumps.

9) Walk for 1 minute to lower your heart rate, or you may move on to step 10.

10) Do 12–16 push-ups using the sofa or on the floor.

11) Pick up your rope, and jump again for 30–45 seconds. You may want to try jumping longer—you can do it!

12) Walk for 2–3 minutes so that your heart rate is down and your breathing becomes more regular.

13) Now lie on your left side on the floor. Your knees should be slightly bent. Keep your foot angled downward.

TIP: Be careful not to turn your knee up toward the ceiling.

Lift and lower your right leg 12–16 times. Without changing sides, bring your right knee into your chest, and then push the leg back out. Repeat 12–16 times. Take that same leg and lift and lower it at a slow even pace 12–16 times.

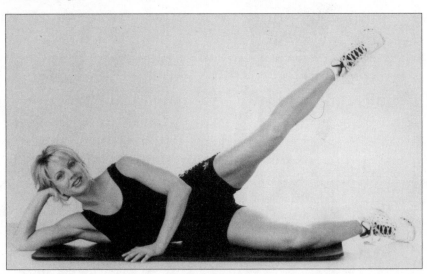

Leg lift

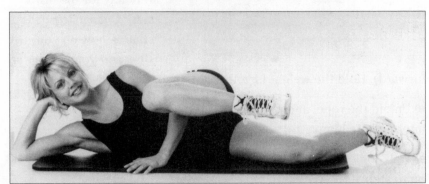

Knee to chest and lengthen out again

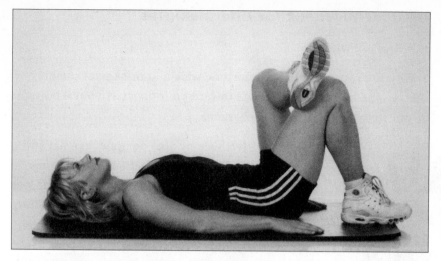

Starting position for stretch

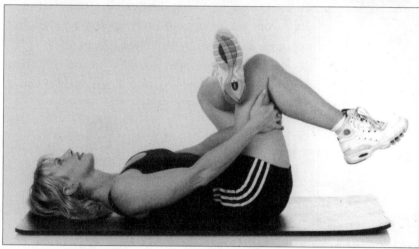

Pulling knee up for more intense stretch

14) Stretch the muscle by lying on your back and bending your knees. Then, place your right ankle over your left quadriceps. Slide your hands through your left leg. To feel this stretch more, pull your leg up in the air.

15) Change sides, and repeat the exercise. (Don't forget that stretch.)

16) Follow the cooldown.

Outdoor Workout for Intermediates

1) Follow the warmup.

2) With the rope folded into quarters, walk at a brisk pace pushing the rope up overhead and down toward your chest as your elbows go out to the side. Repeat 16–20 times.

Rope in eighths

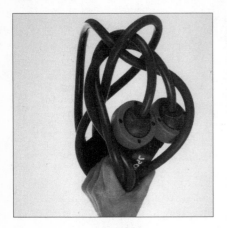

3) Find a curb (this may also be done on a flat surface), and stand a couple of feet away, preparing yourself to lunge into the curb. Stand with your feet together, and lunge forward with your right leg into the curb. You should be on the ball of your foot on your back leg. Your knee should be over your heel on your front leg. Using the muscle strength from your front leg, push your body up so your right leg becomes almost straight. Lower it back to 90 degrees where your heel is over your toe, and then push off to a standing position. It may help if you

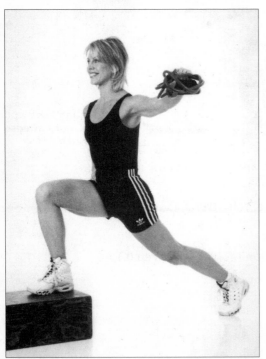

Lunging forward with arm extension

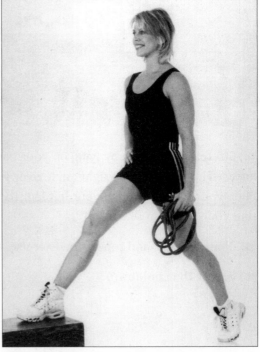

Rising up and lowering arm

say to yourself, "down, halfway up, down, all the way up." Continue to use your arms by folding the rope into eighths and holding it in your left hand. As you lower your body on the lunge, simultaneously raise your arm out to the side. As you rise from the lunge, lower your arm to your side. As you lower into the lunge, raise your arm out to the side. When you push off from the curb, lower your arm back to your side. Repeat on the right side for 8–12 reps.

TIP: Take the time to work this move out. It may seem complicated the first time you read it, but follow the pictures as you read through the exercise. Your buttocks and legs will LOVE you for it.

4) Change legs, and repeat on the left side for 8–12 reps.

5) Unfold the rope, and choose one of the beginner jumps. Jump for 30–45 seconds.

6) Fold the rope back into quarters, and walk for 1 minute to bring your heart rate down.

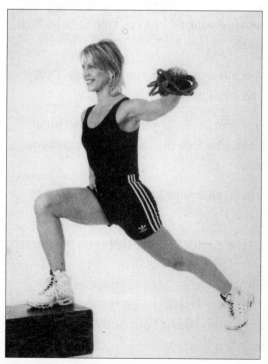

Lowering and extending arm

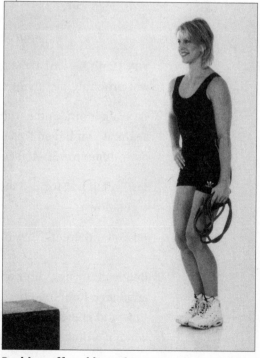

Pushing off and lowering arm

7) Turn sideways, and sidestep down the street—8 steps on one side, face the other side, and sidestep for eight. These 16 steps count as one set. Perform 2–4 sets.

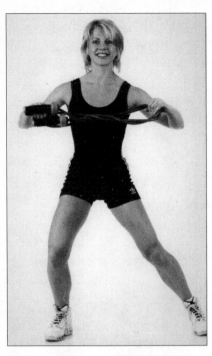

8) Walk to lower your heart rate for 1 minute.

9) Fold the rope in half. Hold your hands over your head using a wide grip on the rope. Squat with your buttocks sitting back. Simultaneously pull the rope down to chest level. As you rise from the squat, push your arms back up overhead. Repeat 12–16 times.

10) Unfold the rope, and choose one of the intermediate jumps. Jump for 30–45 seconds.

11) Walk for 1 minute to lower your heart rate. (This may be a good time to start heading home.)

12) Fold the rope into quarters, and skip—yes, I said "skip"—down the street. You may add more work by moving your arms from side to side. Skip approximately 24 times.

TIP: Don't be embarrassed because you *think* you look silly. People will probably be envious of how happy you look.

13) Walk it out, and catch your breath until you are ready to jump again. If you haven't tried it yet, practice the jumping jack pattern here. Jump for 30–45 seconds.

14) Walk it out for 2–3 minutes to give your heart rate a chance to come down.

15) You did great! Now, follow the cooldown, and be proud of yourself.

Believe it or not, after a while, you will be able to proceed to the advanced jumping chapter. I know you will get there, but take your time and give it a shot when you feel ready. Your body will tell you when it's time to advance your workouts.

CHAPTER 7

JUMP ROPE FOR THE ADVANCED JUMPER

You can modify these advanced workouts to create variation.

Let me remind you that it isn't necessary to master every single advanced jumping pattern to do the advanced workouts. At the simplest level, you may do beginner jumps throughout the whole routine. You may increase the intensity of the workout by varying between intermediate and advanced jumps. There are no steps in between where you are told to walk for 1 minute until the end of the workout, but you may need to before performing the next move. On the other hand, you might want to fold the rope and jog in between if you want a little more challenge from the routine.

Much more balance is required at the advanced level because you work both the arms and legs simultaneously. If you have trouble keeping your balance at this point, you should still try the workout, but hold on to something with one hand and perform the movement with the other. When you change legs on the lunges, change arms, and do the other side instead of the new arm movement.

The advanced workouts have longer jumping portions. In this chapter, I ask you to jump for 1–1$\frac{1}{2}$ minutes. If you jump for 45–60 seconds, that's okay, too. The reverse is also true. By this time, you might find that you love jumping rope and are good at it. You might even decide to do the intermediate and advanced routines, but want to jump for 3–5 minutes instead.

One last thing—you don't have to do any of these workouts alone. Do them with your infant in a stroller outside. Hold on to the stroller for balance during lunges, if necessary. Do them with another mother while the kids are in school. Do them with your husband or wife, boyfriend or girlfriend, before or after work.

Remember, these workouts are designed for every person, every lifestyle, every level of fitness. These workouts are flexible enough to suit you, no matter what schedule you have!

Outdoor Workout for Advanced Jumpers

1) Follow the warmup

2) Fold the rope into quarters, and walk pushing the rope up over-head and bringing it down to chest level for 30 seconds.

3) Find a curb, and face away from it. Put your left foot behind you on the curb and your right foot in front so you are in a lunge position. Lower down, and push up, keeping all the weight on your front heel. Repeat 20 times.

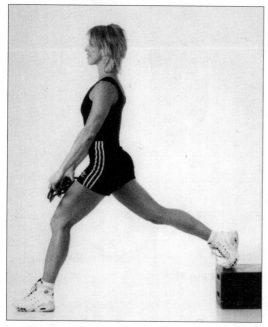

Starting position

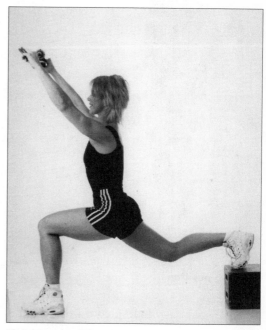

Finishing position

4) Change legs, and repeat on the other side.

5) Now choose a jump, and jump for 30 seconds.

6) Walk it off for 1–1$\frac{1}{2}$ minutes with the rope folded in quarters while pumping your arms back and forth.

7) Now fold the rope in eighths. Lunge forward into the curb, and push off back to a standing position. As you lunge forward, with your right leg, the rope should be in your left hand. Raise your arm to the left side. Repeat 16–20 times.

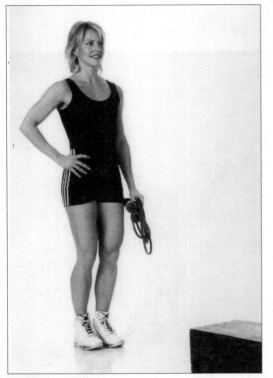

Starting position   **Finishing position**

8) Repeat on the other side.

9) Unfold your rope, and jump for 45–60 seconds.

10) Fold your rope, and sidestep down the street for 8 counts. Change sides for 8 counts. Do 2–4 sets of these.

11) Fold the rope in half, and place the rope overhead, gripping it wide. Perform 20 squats while pulling the rope down in front of you toward your chest and pushing it back up overhead as you rise from the squat.

12) Unfold the rope, and stand in a "ready to jump" position. Jump for 45–60 seconds. (If you have not tried jumping backwards, now may be a good time to do so.)

13) Fold the rope back into quarters, and skip, jog, fast-walk, or do a combo of all three! Do this for 1–1¹/₂ minutes.

TIP: You may get tired soon. Now's the time to head home.

14) Keeping the rope folded in quarters, lunge down the street as if you are taking giant steps, alternating feet. Right foot forward, then left. You may simply hold on to the rope, or you may lift and lower your arms in front of you as you walk. Do 16–20 lunges.

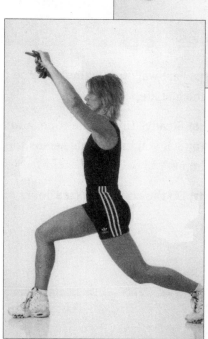

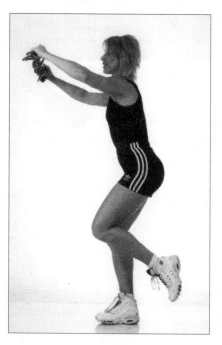

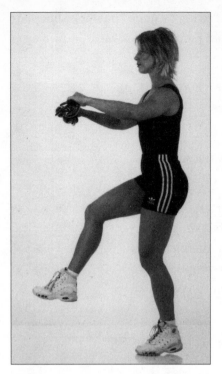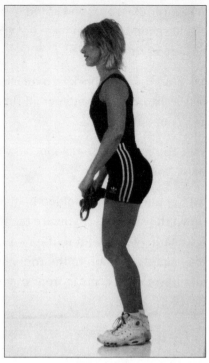

15) Fast-walk for 2 minutes or so (toward home) before completing the last step.

16) Ready? Unfold the rope, and run down the street while jumping rope, if you can. If this seems too advanced, you may jog or fast-walk home.

17) Do the cooldown (outdoors or when you get indoors).

Indoor Workout #1 for the Advanced Jumper

1) Follow the warmup.

2) Unfold the rope, and jump for 45–60 seconds.

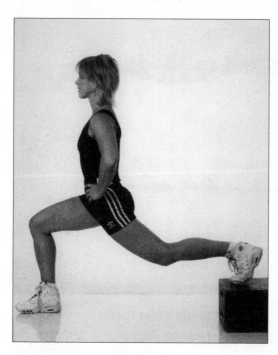

3) Use the steps in your house or apartment, a small stepstool, or, if you have to, pile some books on top of each other (hardcovered preferred) about 8–10 inches high against a wall. Now stand facing away from the step in a lunge position so that the foot of your back leg is on top of the step. Keeping your weight on your front leg, lower your body to where your knee goes no lower than a right angle. Make sure your knee stays aligned over the heel of your foot.

Push your front foot into the floor, and squeeze your buttocks tight to rise back up. Repeat 12–16 times.

4) Change legs, and do the lunges on the other side.

5) Unfold the rope, and jump for 45–60 seconds.

6) Find a chair, the end of a sofa, or a coffee table, if it's strong enough to support your outstretched legs. Do 16–20 triceps dips. You may make them more advanced by elevating your feet.

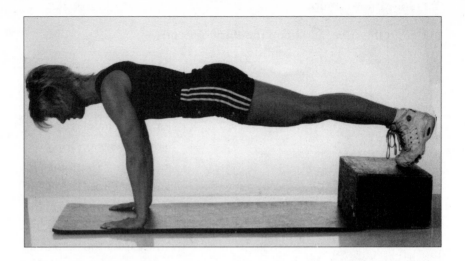

7) Do 12–16 push-ups with your feet raised.

8) Unfold the rope, and jump for 60–90 seconds. Try going backwards if you have not tried that yet.

9) Now stand with your feet apart, slightly wider than your shoulders. Lower your body into a squat position. As you rise from the squat, lift your right leg out to the side. As you lower your leg, lower your body back to the original squat position, and repeat the exercise. Repeat 8–12 times. As you become more skilled at this exercise, you may fold your rope into quarters and place it in your left hand. As your leg lifts out to the right side, your arm lifts laterally to the left side.

10) Change sides so that you squat and lift your left leg to the side. Repeat 8–12 times. Again, the arms are optional.

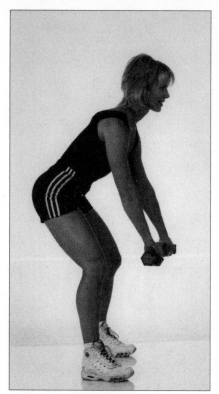

Starting position

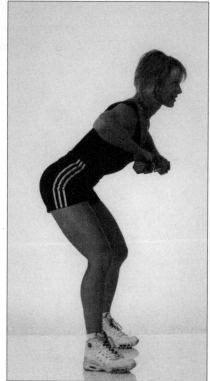

Finishing position

11) You will need a dishtowel and cans or bottles for this next exercise. Use an overhand grip to hold each end of the towel. Keeping your hands in that fixed position, pick up the cans or bottles in each hand. Stand with your feet shoulder-width apart and your knees slightly bent. You should bend over from your hips and not your waist. Extend your arms down, and by squeezing your back, pull your arms up to chest level. Lower your arms back to the floor, and repeat the exercise. Repeat 16–20 times.

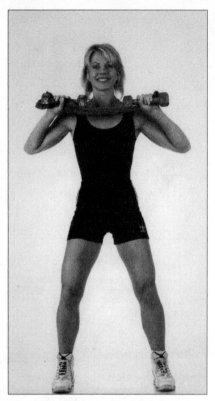 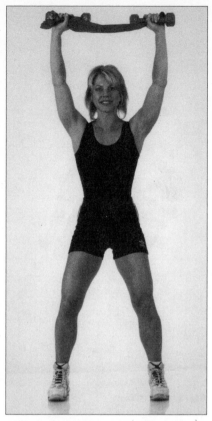

Starting position, shoulder press   **With taut towel, pushing weight overhead**

12) Keeping the weights and towel in the same overhand position, stand up straight with your knees slightly bent. Bring your arms up to shoulder level, and push them up overhead, extending your arms without locking them. Lower them back to shoulder level. Repeat 12–16 times.

13) Pick up the rope, and jump again for 1–1$\frac{1}{2}$ minutes. You may want to try jumping jacks at this point.

14) Walk for 2–3 minutes until your heart rate comes down and you are breathing more regularly.

15) Time for abdominal work! Lie on the floor on your back with your legs straight out and your feet turned out to the side. Place your hands behind your head, and lift and lower your upper body using your abdominals. Do 20 full range and 20 pulses.

16) Follow the cooldown.

Indoor Workout #2 for the Advanced Jumper

1) Follow the warmup.

2) Pick up the rope, and jump for 45–60 seconds.

3) Do 16–20 triceps dips, using a chair or the end of a sofa.

4) Perform 16–20 push-ups on the floor. Remember, when you become more advanced with these, you may go from your knees to your toes.

5) Pick up the rope, and jump for 45–60 seconds.

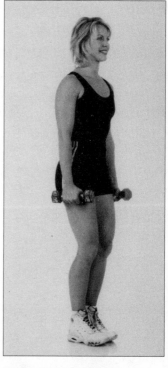

6) Fold the rope into quarters. Down a hallway or clear area in your home, perform walking lunges. This is accomplished by lunging forward with one leg and then bringing the trailing leg to the front for the next lunge. These look like giant steps. Do 16–20 reps. Your arms should be extended in front of you and may rise as high as your forehead and lower to your waist simultaneously with each lunge.

7) Pick up the rope, and jump for 1–1½ minutes, if you can. Don't forget to try jumping backwards. Remember that you may use a combination of jumps to total 1½ minutes.

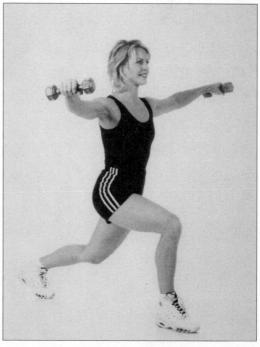

8) Grab hold of cans or bottles for weights. Stand with your feet together. Lunge back with your right leg. Simultaneously lift your arms out to the side to perform lateral raises. As you bring your leg back to standing position, lower your arms back to your side. Repeat 16–20 times.

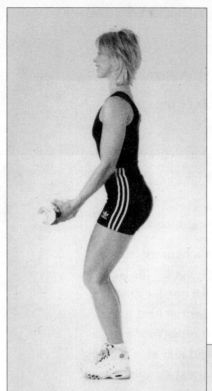

9) Change legs, and repeat on the other side while doing biceps curls with your arms to the side.

10) Jump rope for 1–1$\frac{1}{2}$ minutes.

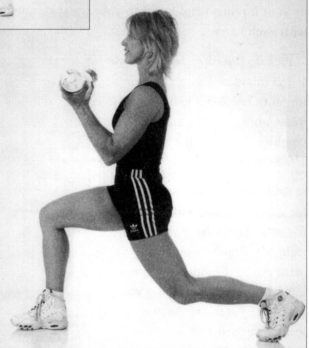

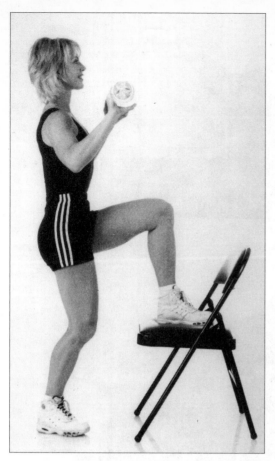

11) Go into the bathroom, and place your right foot on the toilet seat. (Again, make sure the seat is down.) Pressing mostly with your heel into the seat, lift your body up, and extend your left leg behind you. At the same time, you may fold the rope into quarters and raise the rope over your head and then lower it to your chest. You may also use cans or bottles. Repeat 16–20 times.

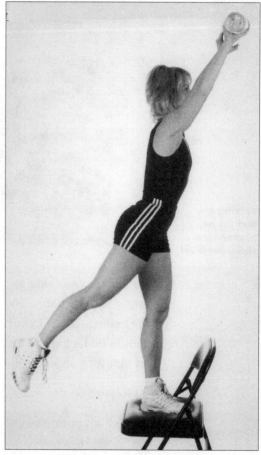

12) Change legs, and perform the previous exercise on your left side. Change your hands to an underhand grip, and reach and pull the folded rope (or your weights) with every lift of your body.

13) Unfold your rope, and jump for 1–1^1/$_2$ minutes.

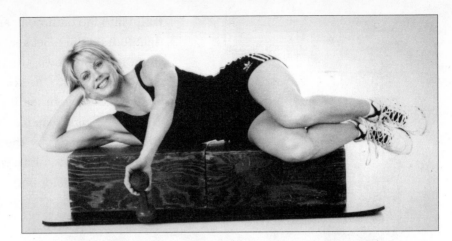

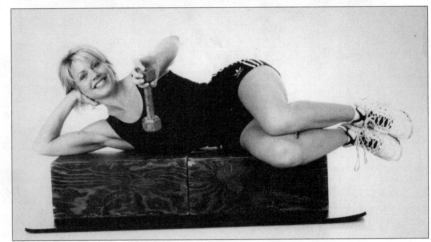

14) Lie on your side on the end of a couch or bed. Hold a can or
bottle in your hand. The end of the can or bottle should be facing
the ceiling. Extend your arm directly out in front of you. Your elbow
should be facing the ceiling. Lower the weight past the bed or couch,
and lift it to shoulder height. Do 12–16 reps.

15) Repeat on the other side.

16) Pick up your rope, and jump for $1–1\frac{1}{2}$ minutes.

17) Walk for 2–3 minutes so that your heart rate comes down and you
feel that you are breathing easier.

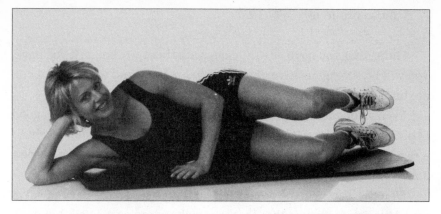

Lifting and
extending leg
in front at
45-degree angle

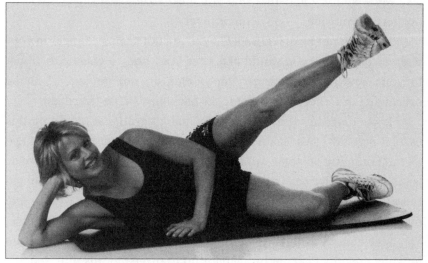

Bending knee
and lowering
to floor

18) Perform side leg lifts on the right side of your body. Lift and lower your leg evenly for 16 reps. Bring your knee into your chest, extend it out, and then lift it up for 16 repetitions. Keeping your foot flexed, extend your leg out in front of you at about a 45-degree angle. Bend your knee, and lower your leg. Lift and extend your leg out in front of you. Bend your knee, and lower your leg. Repeat this 16 times. Perform the outer thigh stretch—lie on your back, and bend your knees. Place your right ankle over your left quadriceps. Slide your hands through your left leg. To feel this stretch more, pull your leg up in the air.

19) Change sides, and repeat on the left side, as well as performing the above outer thigh stretch on the left side.

20) Follow the cooldown.

I am so proud of you!!!

I hope that you have been sticking with these workouts. If you have, you will be seeing positive changes in your body and well-being. Look at yourself in the mirror. You should like what you see.

Even if you are not yet quite at your goal, you should be feeling good about yourself. There is an incredible feeling that comes when you have a regular exercise plan in you life—you become a more confident person in everything that you do.

Exercise can become somewhat addictive—but in a very positive way. My wish for you is that that you make exercise a small, but REGULAR part of your life . . . now and forever.

Please, do not be discouraged if you are not seeing changes in your body as quickly as you would like. Give your body a chance to adjust to your new health pattern. Our bodies do not get out of shape overnight, and, therefore, cannot get back into shape overnight!

I know that almost everyone likes instant gratification, but in this case, it may take two "instants." Exercise takes longer than popping a diet pill or going on some unhealthy crash or starvation diet. Exercise is the only healthy way to get in shape. Many people are unaccustomed to sweating and may be feeling a little sore at first. This takes people out of their comfort and safe zones. Don't be afraid or uncomfortable. You have come this far—don't stop! Every individual is different, and for some, results may not be seen for up to three months. But, remember, ANYTHING that is worthwhile in life takes time—finding the right partner, creating a child, starting your own business.

KEEP IT UP! YOU'RE DOING GREAT!

CHAPTER 8

INTERVAL CIRCUIT TRAINING:
USING THE JUMP ROPE AND MUCH MORE!

By now you have an idea of what interval circuit training is all about and why it is such a great technique to use not only in this program, but in many other exercise programs as well.

Up until now, the jump rope, along with your own body resistance and some weights, has been used throughout the workouts. If at this point you find that you are seriously devoted to exercise (which, if you made it to this chapter, you probably are), then I recommend that you purchase a pair of 3-pound and/or 5-pound weights.

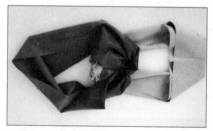

One band over other

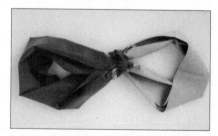

Interlacing them by interlooping

In this chapter, I will also add another piece of equipment—the rubber band or resistive band (also known more generally as resistive tubing). If you have access to a physical therapist, inquire about a resistive band. If not, try your local sporting goods store, or you can even check your local stationery store and purchase a box of extra-large rubber bands.

The workouts in this chapter are by far the most challenging and demanding ones in this book. They require a high level of stamina, balance, and coordination. They may still be done in the privacy of your home, a hotel room, or wherever you may be! Certainly a rubber band and jump rope are easy enough to tuck away in a suitcase—along with this book, of course.

I hope you enjoy the following three workouts! Remember, take it slow. You may have become more advanced and a more serious jumper, but treat your body kindly.

The Ultimate Indoor Interval Workout #1

1) Follow the warmup.

2) Pick up your jump rope, and jump at a moderate pace for 1–2 minutes.

3) Place your rubber band/resistive band around your ankles, and:

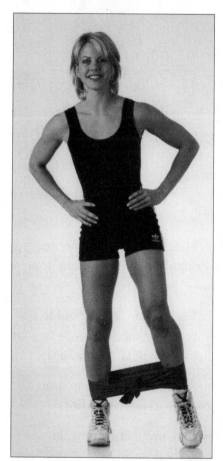 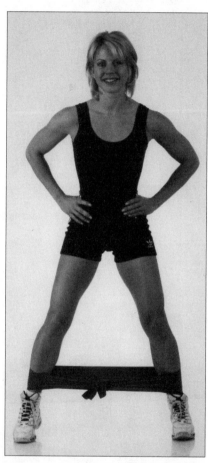

a. Step and touch from side to side. Remember to keep the band taut. Always push from a point of resistance. Repeat 8 times.

b. Take 2 steps to the right and 2 steps to the left. Repeat 8 times.

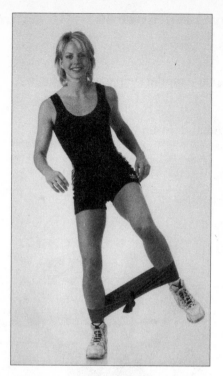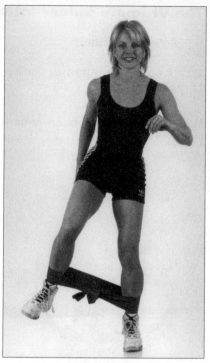

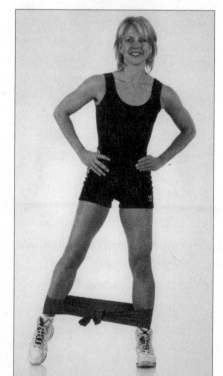

c. March wide. Keep your feet straight. Do not angle out your toes. Repeat 16 times.

d. Push your right leg out to the side for 8 counts. Change to your left leg. Repeat 2 more times.

e. Step and touch again from side to side. Repeat 8 times.

4) Pick up your rope again, and choose from any of the beginner or intermediate jumps. You may perform a combination of any two jumps. Jump for 1–2 minutes.

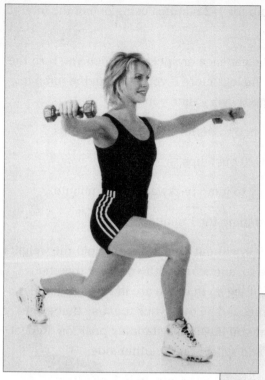

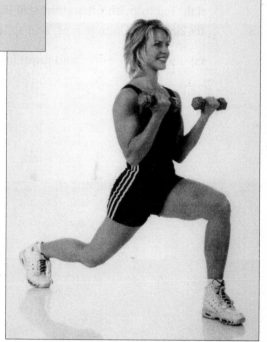

5) Hold the 3- or 5-pound weights in your hands as you stand in a lunge position with your right leg leading. As you lower your body to the floor, raise your arms out to the side. As you rise from the lunge, lower your arms to your side. Repeat for 16–20 times.

6) Change legs. Bring your arms by your side. This time as your body lowers to the floor, bend your elbows to perform biceps curls. Repeat 16–20 times.

TIP: When using weights, never squeeze them tightly.

7) Pick up the rope and jump for 1–2 minutes using one of the intermediate jumps.

TIP: Don't forget to vary the cadence or speed at which you turn the rope. You may emphasize the legs more if you perform the jump in half time and bend your knees every time you *land*.

8) Use a couch, chair, or bench to perform 16–20 triceps dips.

9) On the floor, perform 16–20 push-ups.

10) Pick up the rope, and try to jump backwards for 1 minute.

11) Pick an easier jump, and jump for 1 minute.

12) Do forward lunges with or without your weights. Hold the weights in each hand if you choose to, and stand with your feet together. Step forward with your right leg so that you are in the standard lunge position with your knee in line over your toe. Use that same right leg to push off so that you finish in a standing position. Repeat 16–20 times. Change legs, and repeat on the other side.

13) Pick up the rope, and jump for approximately 2 minutes.

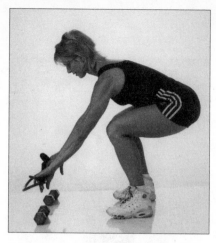

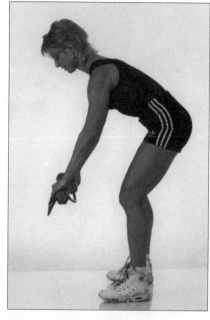

**Starting
position,
upright rows**

14) Fold the rope into quarters, and hold it at the ends using an overhand grip. Pick up your weights, keeping your hands in the same spot. Bend your knees slightly, and bend over slightly from your hip flexor (not your waist). Keeping your shoulders retracted back, extend your arms down toward the floor. By bending your elbows and squeezing your shoulder blades, pull the weights up toward the top of your chest. Lower them to the floor, and repeat the exercise 16–20 times.

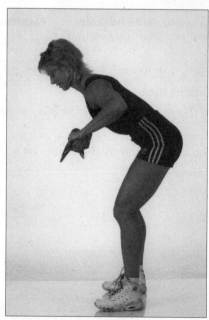

**Finishing position,
upright rows**

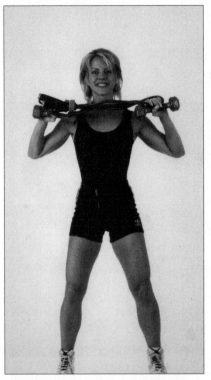 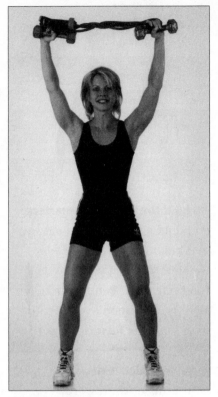

Using a rope or towel to hold arm in fixed position. Starting position

Finishing position

15) Stand up straight with your knees slightly bent, and perform 16–20 shoulder presses.

16) Unfold the rope, and jump for 2–3 minutes using any combination of jumps.

17) Walk for approximately 3 minutes or until your breathing becomes more regular.

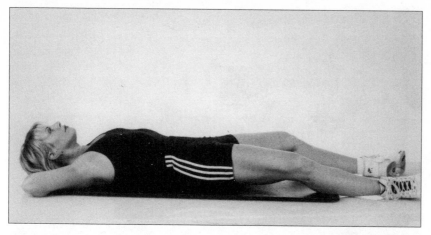

Starting position

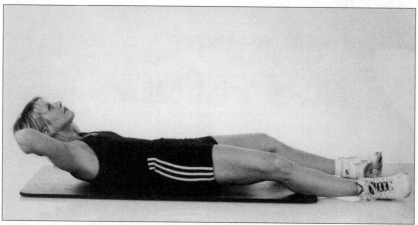

Lifting position

18) Lower your body to the floor with your legs lengthened out and your feet turned out to the side. Place your hands behind your head. Keeping your head in line with your spine, with neck relaxed, contract your abdominal muscles, and lift your upper body. Keeping the contraction on your abdominals, lower your body to the floor without resting, and raise it back up again. Do 16 of these full-range abdominal exercises, and then pulse 16 times. Do 2–3 sets.

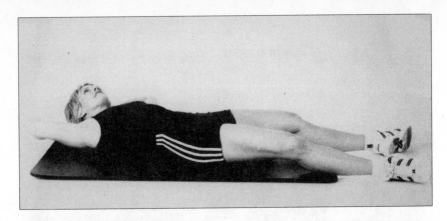

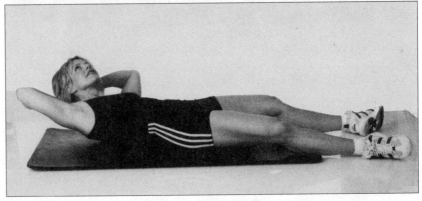

19) Swivel just your upper body over to the right side, and lift toward the left (opposite) side 16 times. Pulse for 16.

20) Change sides, swivel your body to the left side, and lift toward your right side.

21) Go back to the center, and lift and lower your upper body 16 times. You should feel the muscle attachment right around your rib cage.

22) You are now ready to continue with the stretching in the cooldown.

TIP: Remember to drink plenty of water before, during, and after the workout.

The Ultimate Indoor Interval Workout #2

1) Follow the warmup in chapter 4.

2) Jump rope at a moderate pace for 1–2 minutes.

3) Pick up your weights, and stand in a plié position. Your feet should be wide enough so that when you lower your body, your knees are aligned over your heels.

a. Keeping the weights behind you, lower your body by bending your knees. Digging your heels into the floor, rise up and then lower back down again. Keep an even pace. Repeat this 8 times.

b. Next, when you lower your body, pulse 3 times before pushing up. Repeat this 8 times.

c. Lastly, hold in the lowering phase, and pulse for a count of 8 while simultaneously opening your knees wider.

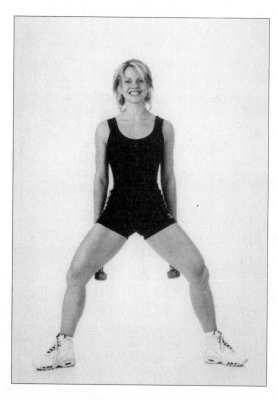 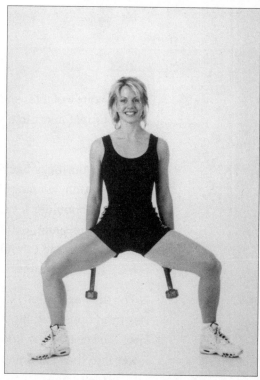

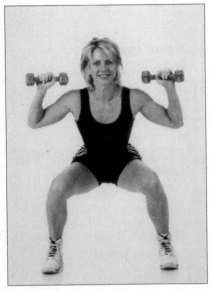

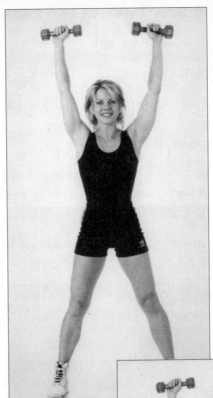

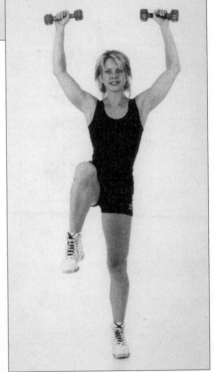

4) Hold your weights, and stand with your feet apart in a squat position.

a. Sit your buttocks back in a squat position, keeping the weights at shoulder level. As you rise from the squat, extend your arms up overhead (shoulder press). Repeat 8 times.

b. For the next set of 12, as you rise from the squat, lift your right knee. Lower it to the floor as you lower into the next squat. Then lift your left knee as you rise from the next squat, and so on.

5) Pick up your rope, and jump for 1–2 minutes.

6) Ready to lie down? Lie on your side at the end of a couch or bed (don't get too comfy!) with one of your weights. Hold the weight with the palm facing down, and lower it past the bed. Lift it to shoulder level, and then slowly lower it to the starting position. Repeat 12–16 times. The weight should be heavy enough to fatigue you. If not, go to a heavier weight. Remember, if you have 3- and 5-pound weights, you may hold one of each instead of buying an 8-pound weight.

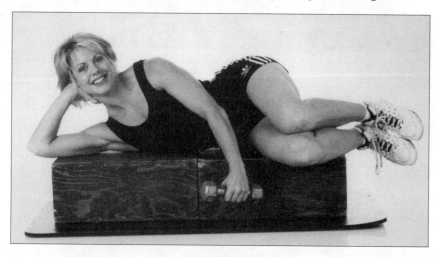

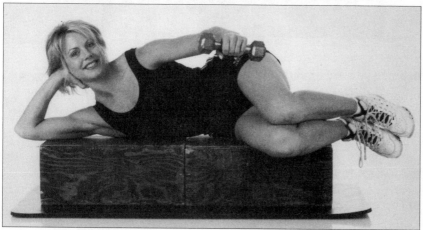

7) Flip over to the other side, and repeat the same exercise 12–16 times.

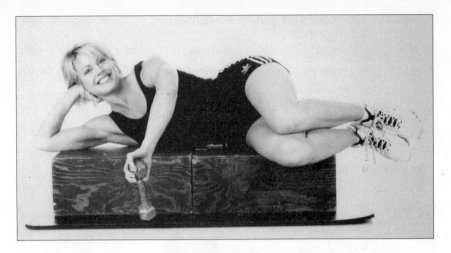

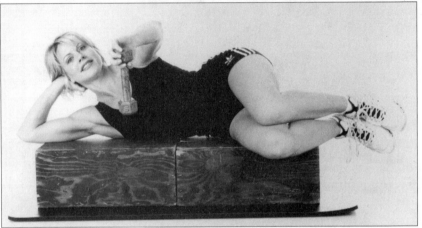

8) Since you are already in this position, flip back again to the other side. Hold the weight so that the end of the weight is facing the ceiling. Although your elbow is bent, your arm should be extended out at shoulder level or slightly lower. Lower the weight past the bed, and lift it to shoulder level. Slowly lower it again. Repeat 12–16 times.

9) Flip over to the other side, and repeat the same exercise 12–16 times.

10) Stand up, and jump rope for approximately 2 minutes. (Any jumping pattern is okay.)

11) Take out the rubber band/resistive band, and place it around your ankles. Keeping the band taut at all times:

a. Step and touch from side to side 8 times.

b. Take 2 steps to the right and 2 steps to the left. Repeat 8 times. Remember, do not angle out your toes.

c. Keeping your feet as wide as possible, march wide 12 times.

d. Lift your heels back and slightly angled out to the side 8 times.

e. Lift your heels back twice on each side 8 times.

f. Step and touch from side to side 8 times.

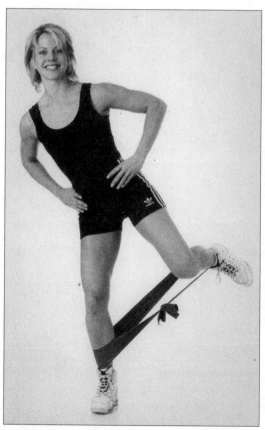
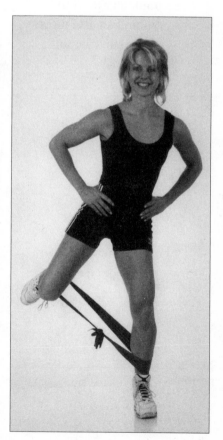

Keeping legs wide enough apart so band is taut

12) Using a chair, do 16–20 triceps dips. If these become easy, you should make them more challenging by extending your legs out on the floor or even more so by elevating your legs on another chair.

13) Jump rope for 2 minutes. Try going backwards.

14) Stand in a lunge position with your left leg forward and your right leg back. You may hold on to weights in each hand. Lower your body to the floor only as low as where your knee is at a right angle. As you rise from the lunge, push your heel into the floor, and lift your back leg behind you. As you lower your leg back down, bend your front knee again, readying yourself for the next lift. Repeat 12–16 times. You may increase the difficulty level by adding an arm movement such as pull backs.

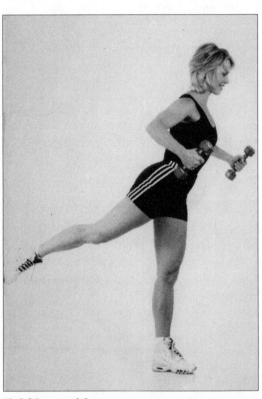

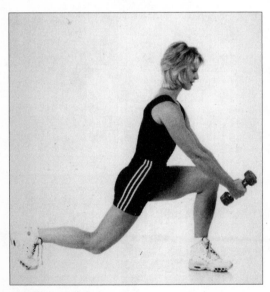

Starting position

Finishing position

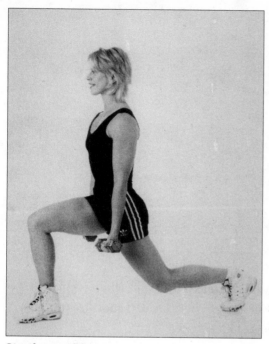

Starting position

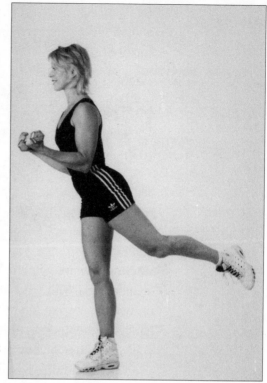

Finishing position

15) Change legs, and repeat on the other side 12–16 times. You may perform biceps curls simultaneously if you would like an arm exercise.

16) Jump rope for approximately 1–2 minutes.

17) Walk around your house or apartment for 2–3 minutes or until you are breathing more regularly. You are approaching the end of the workout so it is important for your heart rate to come down.

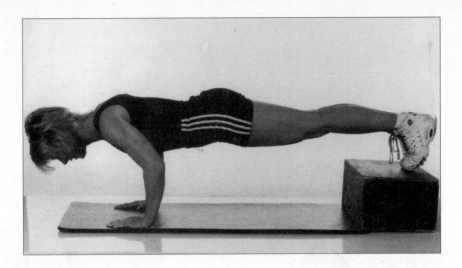

18) Now, you are going to do 12–16 push-ups one of two ways. You may do them with your legs extended and your upper body elevated, or if you feel up to it, you may elevate your legs and place your hands on the floor. In either case, make sure that when you lower your upper body, your hands are at chest level. If they are too high, you will be working your shoulders.

19) Follow the cooldown starting from step 2.

The Ultimate Outdoor Interval Workout

1) Follow the warmup in chapter 4.

2) Fold the rope into quarters, and lift and lower the rope from chest level up overhead and back 20 times.

3) Sidestep down the street for 8 counts, and then change to the other side for 8 counts. This is one set. Perform 4–6 sets.

4) Unfold your rope, and jump for 1–2 minutes.

5) Fold the rope into quarters, and find a curb. Stand with your back facing away from the curb in a lunge position so that your back foot is elevated on the curb. As you lower your body, simultaneously extend and lift your arms up and in front of you. As you raise your body from the lunge, lower your arms. Repeat 16–20 times.

6) As you change legs, change your hands to an underhand grip on the rope. Lower your body while your arms extend slightly up and out. As you rise from the lunge, pull them down and into your side. Repeat 16–20 times.

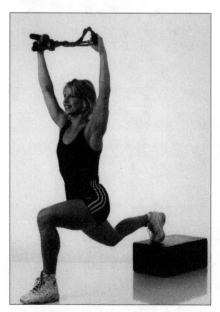 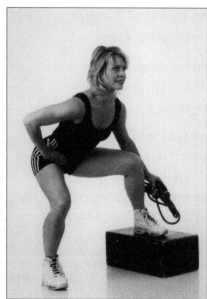

7) Jump rope backwards for 1–2 minutes.

8) Again fold the rope into quarters, and skip down the street for approximately 50 skips.

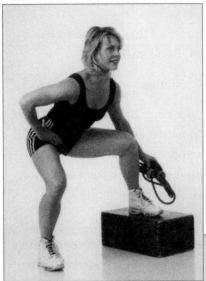

Starting position

9) Find another curb, and, in a squat position, place your left foot on it. Fold the rope in eighths, and place it in your left hand. Sit back into the squat. Rise from the squat, and lift the leg that is on the street (right leg) out to the side. Simultaneously, keep your palm facing down, and lift your left arm out to the side. Repeat 16–20 times.

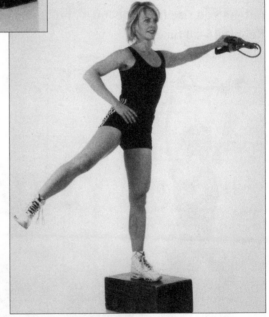

Finishing position

10) Repeat 16–20 times on the other side.

11) Unfold your rope, and jump for approximately 2 minutes.

12) Fold the rope into quarters, and lunge down the street. You may want to set a goal of doing between 16 and 24 lunges.

13) This step may be done anytime in the workout since everybody's neighborhood is different. If you see a bench in a park or some type of wall that is no higher than your hips, use it to get in 16–20 triceps dips.

14) Unfold your rope, and run and jump simultaneously down the street. If you are in a neighborhood with blocks, do this for a block, and then fast-walk for a block, run and jump for a block, and then fast-walk for a block. Use your discretion.

15) Walk or jog for about 1 minute to lower your heart rate for the next set of lunges.

16) You will now combine two lunges into one. Stand with your feet together facing the curb. Lunge into the curb with your left leg. Lower your body so your front knee stays over your heel and bends no more than 90 degrees. By driving your heel into the curb, push your body back up into a standing position. Now lunge back (using the same right leg) behind you, and come back up to standing position. As you get better at this move, you will not need to stand in between, but rather just touch the street with your toe to stay aligned. The combination of both lunges counts as one. Do 10–12 reps.

17) Change legs, and repeat 10–12 repetitions on the other side.

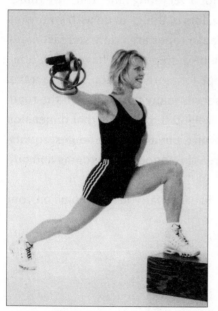 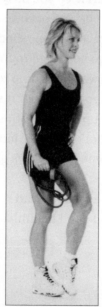 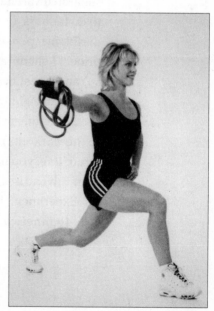

Left leg lunge forward; left leg coming back to center position; left leg lunge backward

By now you should be nearing your house or starting point.

18) To get back home, you may jog, jump rope, fast-walk, or do a combination of all three!

19) Follow cooldown step 1. Before you continue on with step 2, do 16–20 push-ups, using any one of the previously discussed methods.

20) Finish the cooldown.

How do you feel? I hope that these routines have provided you with enough variation for you to avoid boredom. Being bored should not even enter your mind, since these workouts can be modified each time you do them (different jumps, different weights, whatever suits your fancy). The time should fly by since you are constantly changing activities and moving to the next exercise. That is the beauty of interval circuit training.

So, you say to yourself, NOW WHAT?! If you have reached this point in the book, I hope that you have done all the workouts and that the suggested variations keep you busy for a very long time. You have things to do indoors and out, and of course, lots of things to do with your wonderful, inexpensive jump rope. Because ropes are really so reasonably priced, I encourage you to go to the next step (if you haven't yet done so) and invest in a weighted jump rope for more variation. I like to travel with my weighted rope because it serves many purposes. On the road, I use it to tone my upper body (the weighted rope adds that dimension to the workouts) not only while jumping, but also in the lunges, squats, stretching, you name it. And, it is great for indoor hotel rooms and outdoor adventures.

Experiment, be creative, and realize how far you have come on your road to fitness and good health.

CHAPTER 9

INVOLVING FRIENDS AND FAMILY

All the workouts in this book may be done with a partner. In this chapter, I will explore additional ways that you can incorporate other people into your new healthy lifestyle. By involving your friends and family, you establish immediate motivation for yourself. Excuses like "I have no time to exercise because I have to watch my kids" don't exist anymore, since I will show you creative ways to work out while you are WITH your kids. Other excuses like "my spouse doesn't like to work out, and I don't want to take quality time away from us" also don't exist anymore. Also, what is better than working out with a friend or mate whom you can support and who can support you in making the time and effort for exercise?

Time with Infants and Toddlers

Moms can get together and wheel their strollers intermittently with jumping rope for 15–30 seconds, then continuing to walk with the stroller. If you have kids ages three or up, you can give them their own jump rope to occupy them while you jump. There are many ropes on the market today that are perfect for kids. They have eye-popping colors, handles that play music, you name it. Kids are truly thrilled to be doing the same thing that their mom or dad are doing. They mimic, and what a great role model you can be to your children by showing them that exercise is a regular and important part of your life. You will be giving your family a wonderful gift by encouraging them to exercise.

I have a young daughter, and there were many times when I didn't have a baby-sitter, but was still determined to exercise. I would take her to the park across the street from our home and give her a pink jump rope. Most kids this young cannot jump rope yet. So I jumped rope while my daughter tried to turn it. She also tried to jump and play on her own. Of course, my "workout" was interrupted by her questions and her need for guidance and attention, but she looked at our time in the park together as true quality time. Just the two of us playing (she didn't see it as a workout!) was great for her and me, too. We played follow-the-leader, and I taught her how to sidestep, skip, and when I did lunges while walking, she took fun giant steps. She had a blast. Another benefit was that she would be exhausted by seven on those nights and would go to bed early.

You can also take a ball (kick ball, soccer ball, etc.) outside while you do this. Kids can do any number of things with a ball. You can even kick the ball back and forth to each other, and while she rests or chases after it, you can jump.

Another great idea, which has worked wonderfully for my daughter and me, is to skip and jump rope next to her while she rides her bicycle. You don't have to jump the whole time. Let her ride the bike, and you can race-walk, jog, or jump. Be creative. Have fun. If you have forgotten how, let your child show you!

Age Five and Up

As kids get a little older, usually around age five, they are able to become more agile at jumping. There are many jumps that the two of you can do together. Here are my favorites.

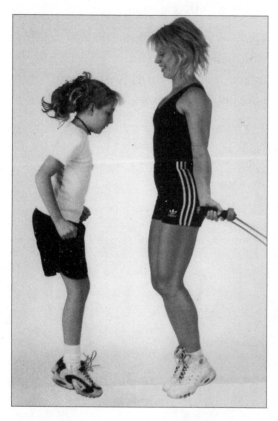

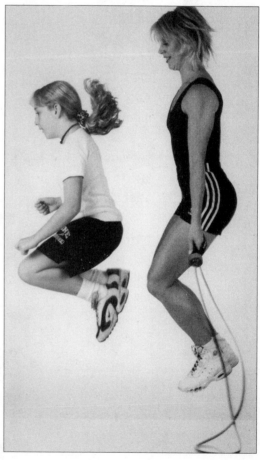

1) Face each other, and jump together using one rope.

2) Face in the same direction, and jump rope.

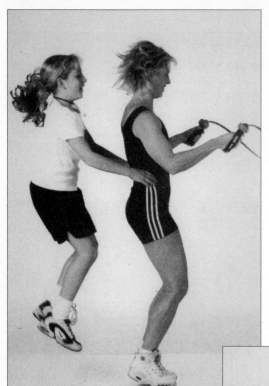

3) Try jumping backwards together with one rope.

4) Involve a third person (maybe a husband, wife, friend, or your child's friend), and take turns twirling and jumping with the rope.

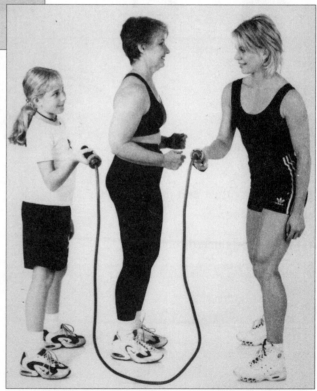

5) Play the game "snake" (perhaps your remember this from when you were a kid). Wiggle the rope back and forth, and have the person jump over it. It is a good movement change.

6) Twirl the rope around and have one, two, or more people jump over the rope. Take turns twirling.

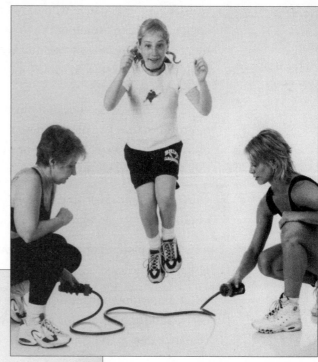

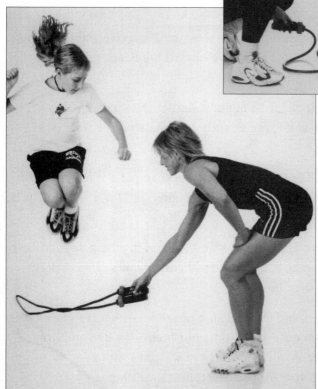

Pals and Partners

Exercising with another adult is also extremely beneficial and is another kind of motivation in your workout program. I really enjoy working out with someone because while I am doing the exercise, I am also being social. This takes some of the pressure and focus off the exercise, and the time goes by much more quickly. My friends and I have solved world problems on the streets while jumping rope and walking around Bergen County, New Jersey!

Every one of the workouts in this book can be done with a partner or group so that you have someone else to motivate you. Here are some of my favorite ways for pairs or groups to make the TIME to work out together. So, grab your mate's hand, or call a friend, and get started.

• Invite a friend over to exercise (or to go for a walk) instead of talking on the telephone for 20 or 30 minutes.

• Workout instead of a dinner or movie date with your boyfriend/girlfriend/spouse.

• Get a morning baby-sitter on the weekend, exercise with your mate early, and then go out for a healthy reward breakfast. (Who says romance needs to be at night?)

• Set your alarm clock for 25 minutes earlier than usual—before the kids wake up—and exercise with your mate on the floor of your bedroom or living room.

• Prepare and eat dinner 20 minutes later than usual a few nights a week, and take your mate (and even the kids) out for a workout or a long, brisk walk.

• Make a lunch-date appointment, and instead of eating at your desk or skipping lunch, take a 25-minute walk or do one of the workouts with a friend, and then have lunch.

• When meeting a friend for a meal, if possible, pick a restaurant that is about a 15-minute walk from your home. Walk to and from your social appointment (30 minutes of walking) with or without the person you are meeting for breakfast, lunch, or dinner.

• While you and your friend/mate are watching a video, do squats, lunges, and ab work from this book in front of the television.

• On a cold and snowy or rainy day, go to your local shopping mall with a friend. Before you shop, browse, or eat, make a deal with each other that you will briskly walk around the mall (a couple of "laps") together before you spend any money.

Assisting Your Partner

If you are choosing to do the workouts in this book with someone, here are a few ways that you can physically assist your partner.

1) HAMSTRING STRETCH: The true test of a flexible hamstring is when the leg that is being stretched is perpendicular to the floor while the resting leg is extended on the floor. You may start by keeping the resting leg bent at the knee. Have your partner gently bring the leg to be stretched up toward a perpendicular position to the floor. Your partner must communicate with you when to stop and hold. At that point, hold your partner's leg, and have him/her push into you gently while you hold steady. You should both be pushing into each other with equal force. Your partner's leg is actually stretching. Please make sure you communicate with each other about when to release.

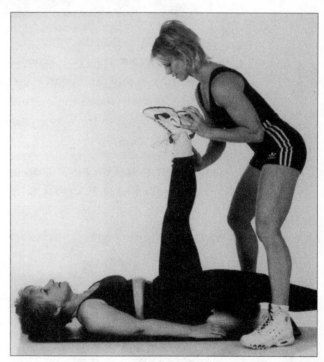

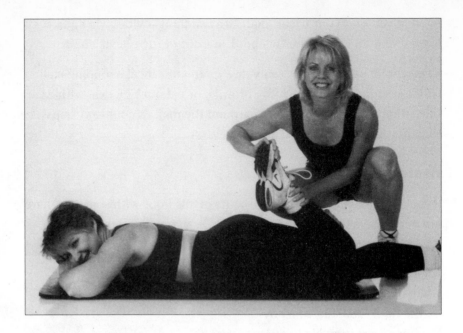

2) QUADRICEPS STRETCH: Have your partner lie on his/her stomach. Take his/her foot, and bend it up toward his/her buttock. A flexible quadriceps will touch the buttock. Remember to do this slowly and gently so as not to hurt your partner. Think of it as an exercise in communication.

3) OUTER THIGH OR ABDUCTOR STRETCH: Cross your partner's right foot over his/her left knee. Lift the left knee, and gently push it

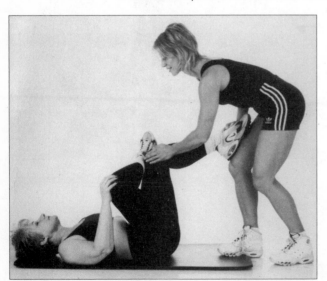

toward your partner's chest. Simultaneously pull his/her right knee toward you. Again, these are equal and opposite forces that will allow the muscle to stretch. Your partner should communicate to you to "push more or lighten up." Change legs and repeat on the other side.

4) ARM STRETCH: Stand with your arms raised over your head and your palms facing each other. Gently press your head down through your shoulders. You should feel this stretch throughout your whole arm, but mostly under your arms.

5) SIT DOWN WITH YOUR PARTNER,
facing each other, legs open in a V-shape, with the bottom of your feet touching the bottom of your partner's feet. Reach for each other's hands, keeping your back as straight as possible and your buttocks on the floor. Communicate with each other and gently pull your partner toward you, until he/she feels a maximum stretch without any pain. Hold the stretch, and instruct your partner to squeeze his/her legs against yours. Hold that position for 15–20 seconds. Slowly release. Your partner now may be able to stretch his/her legs slightly wider. Do the stretch again. Switch roles, and let your partner pull you.

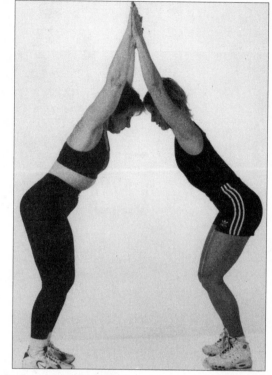

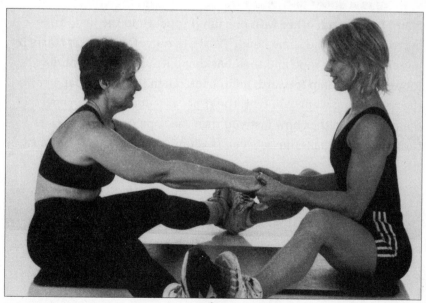

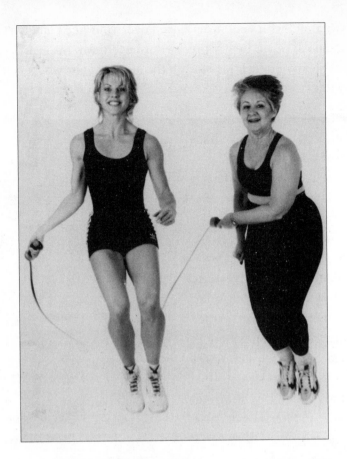

6) HERE IS A JUMP FOR THE TWO OF YOU to do together:
Stand facing each other with one jump rope. Hold the jump rope
mirror image in the same hand. Twirl the rope. One person starts by
jumping into the rope and then backing out. The movement may be
thought of as jump forward, jump back. Then have your partner do
the same thing while you twirl the rope. You decide on the speed of
the jumps by either how fast you turn the rope or the number of
turns the rope makes in between the jumps.

CHAPTER 10

CONCLUSION

Now that you have tried many (maybe ALL!) of the workouts in this book, you might be saying to yourself, "Great, I loved it! I am going to do this every day!" Right? Wrong!

People tend to set themselves up for failure by making fierce demands on themselves and establishing unrealistic goals. Please, don't do this to yourself with exercise.

One of the ways to stay motivated is to allow yourself some freedom and not make exercise a chore. It is much more realistic and reasonable to say, "This wasn't too bad. I can do this. I will set aside time three days a week." Believe me, when you are ready, you will realize how good exercise makes you feel about so many different things in your life and you will find ways to fit it three times a week into your schedule (and possibly increase your workouts to four or more times a week without any pressure).

For people with kids, it may be easier to exercise on Saturday and Sunday when your spouse is home to help out. Then, if you exercised just one more time during the week, that makes three workouts! Or, maybe weekends are not as convenient, and Monday, Wednesday, and Friday sound better; or Monday, Tuesday, and Thursday; or Tuesday, Thursday, and Friday—you get the point. You might prefer the morning or evening or lunchtime. Remember, THERE ARE NO RULES. Exercising only THREE TIMES A WEEK is an amazing commitment and accomplishment.

If you cannot even imagine cramming one more thing into your schedule and feel it is completely unrealistic to make time for three workouts, then take out your appointment book and write "EXERCISE" in three different days of the week. It is an important appointment that you simply CANNOT break. You will surprise yourself when you see that you can actually do this.

Unfortunately, we want immediate gratification and hope for immediate results. That is why diet pills, crash diets, cellulite cream, and herbal wraps exist. You may think you're getting instant results, but they are VERY unhealthy or simply untrue in their claims, and at best, offer only temporary results.

The plain, honest truth is that to make a change in yourself, you have to make a change in yourself! People limit themselves by what they believe they can and cannot do. Try to break out of that mind-set. Step out of the safe boundaries in which you have lived. Go back to the beginning of this book, and look at the list of what exercise can do for you. It bears repeating that it takes time to get out of shape, so it naturally follows that it takes time to get into shape.

Don't have unrealistic expectations. If you were a great jump roper or terrific athlete when you were a child, and it has been twenty-five years since you've done any exercise, please don't think you're going to pick up where you left off.

Most of all, remember that good things take time. When you commit to an exercise program for life, then you are committing to a better life. The long term is what this is about. As you get older and face the many good and bad things that life will throw your way, you want to have a strong and healthy body, as well as a clear mind. A commitment to exercise and good health will do that for you, and it will make you a happier, healthier, stronger, more confident human being.

Trust me. I've seen it happen to hundreds of people, and I know that it can happen to you.

Here's to your health!

THE END!

Beginner Indoor Workout #1

1) warmup

2) 8–12 squats

3) jump rope, 15–30 seconds

4) push-ups, 16 reps

5) lateral raises (shoulder raises), 12–16 reps

6) jump rope, 15–30 seconds

7) backward lunges, 8–12 reps (right leg)

8) backward lunges, 8–12 reps (left leg)

9) jump rope, 15–30 seconds

10) cooldown

Beginner Indoor Workout #2

1) warmup

2) 8–12 squats

3) jump rope, 15–30 seconds

4) alternating knee lifts

5) forward lunges, 8–12 reps (right leg)

6) forward lunges, 8–12 reps (left leg)

7) jump rope, 15–30 seconds

8) lateral raises, 12–16 reps

9) shoulder presses, 12–16 reps

10) jump rope, 15–30 seconds

11) side leg lifts (right leg), 12–16 reps

12) side leg lifts (left leg), 12–16 reps

13) cooldown

Beginner Outdoor Workout

1) warmup

2) shoulder presses with rope in quarters while walking

3) walk while lifting and lowering arms

4) jump rope, 15–30 seconds

5) walk, 1 minute

6) 8–12 squats

7) jump rope, 15–30 seconds

8) stationary lunges, 8–12 reps (right leg)

9) stationary lunges, 8–12 reps (left leg)

10) jump rope, 15–30 seconds

11) walk, 2–3 minutes

12) cooldown

Intermediate Indoor Workout #1

1) warmup

2) jump rope, 30–45 seconds

3) walk, 1 minute

4) squat to right, squat to left, repeat 8 times

5) lateral raises, 12–16 reps

6) jump rope, 30–45 seconds

7) walk, 1 minute

8) triceps dips, 8–12 reps

9) push-ups, 12–16 reps

10) jump rope, try for 1 minute

11) walk, 1 minute

12) buttocks toner in bathroom (right leg), 12–16 reps

13) buttocks toner in bathroom (left leg), 12–16 reps

14) jump rope, 30–45 seconds

15) walk until heart rate comes down

16) abdominal exercises—16 full range—16 pulses

17) cooldown

Intermediate Indoor Workout #2

1) warmup

2) fold rope in half, squat pulsing 3 times, rise

3) jump rope, 30–45 seconds

4) walk, 1 minute

5) triceps dips, 12–16 reps

6) stationary lunges with lateral raise
(right leg, left arm), 8–12 reps

7) stationary lunges with lateral raise
(left leg, right arm), 8–12 reps

8) jump rope, 30–45 seconds

9) walk, 1 minute

10) 12–16 push-ups

11) jump rope, 30–45 seconds

12) walk, 2–3 minutes

13) leg lifts, 12–16 reps; knee into chest, 12–16

14) stretch

15) change sides

16) stretch

17) cooldown

Intermediate Outdoor Workout

1) warmup

2) fold rope in quarters and walk pushing arms overhead

3) down/halfway up/down/all the way up, lunges into curb with lateral raises, rope in eighths (right leg, left arm)

4) repeat on other side (left leg, right arm)

5) jump rope, 30–45 seconds

6) fold rope in quarters, and walk 1 minute

7) sidestep down street

8) walk, 1 minute

9) squat with "lat pulldowns," 12–16 reps

10) jump rope, 30–45 seconds

11) walk, 1 minute

12) rope in quarters, skip 24 times down street

13) walk until ready to jump, jump rope 30–45 seconds

14) walk, 2–3 minutes

15) cooldown

Advanced Outdoor Workout

1) warmup

2) fold rope in quarters, push rope overhead

3) "trailing leg on curb" lunges (right leg), 20 reps

4) "trailing leg on curb" lunges (left leg), 20 reps

5) jump rope, 30 seconds

6) walk, $1-1^1/_2$ minutes

7) rope into eighths, lateral raise (left arm), lunge into curb (right leg), 16–20 reps

8) change sides and repeat, 16–20 reps

9) jump rope, 45–60 seconds

10) sidestep down street, 8 counts each side, 2–4 sets

11) 20 squats with "lat pulldowns"

12) jump rope, 45–60 seconds

13) skip, jog, or fast-walk down street, $1-1^1/_2$ minutes

14) lunge down street, 16–20 reps

15) fast-walk toward home 2 minutes

16) run down street while jumping

17) cooldown

Advanced Indoor Workout #1

1) warmup
2) jump rope, 45–60 seconds
3) trailing leg lunges (right leg), 12—16 reps
4) repeat on other side
5) jump rope, 45–60 seconds
6) 16–20 triceps dips
7) 12-16 push-ups
8) jump rope, 1–1$^1/_2$ minutes
9) squat, lift (right leg) as you rise, left arm lifts laterally, 8–12 reps
10) repeat on other side (left leg, right arm)
11) upright rows, 16–20 reps
12) shoulder presses, 12–16 reps
13) jump rope, 1–1$^1/_2$ minutes
14) walk, 2–3 minutes
15) 20 full-range sit-ups, 20 pulses
16) cooldown

Advanced Indoor Workout #2

1) warmup

2) jump rope, 45–60 seconds

3) 16–20 triceps dips

4) 16–20 push-ups

5) jump rope, 45–60 seconds

6) walking lunges, 16–20 reps

7) jump rope, 1–1$^{1}/_{2}$ minutes

8) backward lunges (right leg) with lateral raises, 16–20 reps

9) backward lunges (left leg) with biceps curls, 16–20 reps

10) jump rope, 1–1$^{1}/_{2}$ minutes

11) buttocks toner in bathroom (right leg) with shoulder press, 16–20 reps

12) buttocks toner in bathroom (left leg) with reach and pull for upper body, 16–20 reps

13) jump rope, 1–1$^{1}/_{2}$ minutes

14) posterior deltoid (right arm), 12–16 reps

15) change sides and repeat

16) jump rope, 1–1$^{1}/_{2}$ minutes

17) walk, 2–3 minutes

18) side leg lifts (right leg), 16 reps
knee into chest, 16 reps
lift, extend, and lower, 16 reps

19) repeat on other side

20) cooldown

Ultimate Interval Circuit Indoor Workout #1

1) warmup

2) jump rope, 1–2 minutes

3) rubber band—step, touch side to side, 8 reps

    —2 steps right, 2 steps left, 8 reps

    —march wide, 16 reps

    —right leg touch side, left leg touch side, 3 reps

    —step and touch, 8 reps

4) jump rope, 1–2 minutes

5) standing lunges with lateral raises (right leg), 16–20 reps

6) standing lunges with biceps curls (left leg), 16–20 reps

7) jump rope, 1–2 minutes

8) triceps dips, 16–20 reps

9) push-ups, 6–20 reps

10) jump rope backwards, 1 minute

11) pick another jump, jump rope, 1 minute

12) forward lunges, with or without weights, 16–20 reps

13) repeat on other side

14) jump rope, 2 minutes

15) upright rows, 16–20 reps

16) shoulder presses, 16–20 reps

17) jump rope, 2–3 minutes

18) walk, 2–3 minutes

19) abdominals—16 full range, 2–3 sets

    —16 pulse, 2–3 sets

20) swivel to side—16 full range, 2–3 sets

    —16 pulse, 2–3 sets

21) change sides and repeat

22) go back to center and left, 16 reps

23) cooldown

Ultimate Interval Circuit Indoor Workout #2

1) warmup

2) jump rope, 1–2 minutes

3) plié for 8 reps

4) plié and pulse for 3 then rise

5) plié and hold, press knees open wider

6) squat with shoulder press, 8 reps

7) squat with knee lifts and shoulder press, 12 reps

8) jump rope, 1–2 minutes

9) arm lateral raises, 12–16 reps

10) repeat on other side

11) posterior deltoid, 12–16 reps

12) repeat on other side

13) jump rope, 2 minutes

14) rubber band—step and touch, 8 reps

—2 steps right, 2 steps left, 8 reps

—march wide, 12 reps

—hamstring curls, 8 reps each side

—step and touch, 8 reps

15) triceps dips, 16–20 reps

16) jump rope backwards, 2 minutes

17) trailing leg lift lunge with pullbacks, 12–16 reps

18) trailing leg lift lunge with biceps curls, 12–16 reps

19) jump rope, 1–2 minutes

20) walk, 2–3 minutes

21) 12–16 push-ups with elevated legs

22) cooldown

Ultimate Interval Circuit Outdoor Workout

1) warmup

2) push rope folded in quarters up overhead

3) sidestep, 4–6 sets

4) jump rope, 1–2 minutes

5) trailing leg lunge with arm extension, 16–20 reps

6) repeat on other side with underhanded grip and pull, 16–20 reps

7) jump rope, 1–2 minutes

8) skip 50 times down street

9) lateral lift with squat, leg lift, 16–20 reps

10) change sides and repeat, 16–20 reps

11) jump rope, 2 minutes

12) lunge down street, 16–24 reps

13) triceps dips, 16–20 dips

14) run down street jumping rope

15) walk or jog, 1 minute

16) combination lunges (forward and back), 10–12 reps

17) change sides and repeat

18) jog, jump rope, or fast-walk home

19) walk 2–3 minutes

20) push-ups, 16–20 reps

21) cooldown

SELECTED BIBLIOGRAPHY

Botermans, Jack et al., *The World of Games: Their Origin and History* (New York & Oxford: Facts on File, 1989).

Church, Matt, "Games Trainers Play," *IDEA Personal Trainer* (October 19, 1996): 20-26.

Goldstein, Robert L., ed., *Aerobics Instructor Manual* (San Diego, CA: American Council on Exercise & Boston: Reebok University Press, 1993).

Kalbfleisch, Susan, *JUMP! The New Jump Rope Book* (New York: William Morrow & Company, 1985).

Kravitz, Len, "Circuits and Intervals," *IDEA Today* (January 1996): 33–38.

LaForge, Ralph, "Interval Exercise," *IDEA Personal Trainer* (November/December 1994): 19–24.

Solis, Ken, *Ropics: The Next Jump Forward in Fitness* (Champaign, IL: Leisure Press, 1992).